THE
CHAKRA SYSTEM
— of —
MOUNT DESERT
ISLAND

THE CHAKRA SYSTEM

_of_

MOUNT DESERT ISLAND

A Guidebook

P. Chris Kaiser

North Atlantic Books • Berkeley, California

The Chakra System of Mount Desert Island

Published by
North Atlantic Books
P.O. Box 12327, Berkeley, California 94712

Cover and book design by Nancy Koerner

Photos on pages 3, 5, 17, 27, 48, 50, 53, 73, 79, 85, 103, 105, 108, 114, 121, and 125 by Chris Kaiser. Photos on pages v, xi, 13, 45, 56, 58, 105, and 127 courtesy Raymond Strout. Postcard reproductions on pages 14 and 31 courtesy Island Images. Satellite views on pages 95 through 101 from U.S. Geological Survey, Eros Data Center. Photos on pages 69 and 113 by Earl Brechlin. Photo on page 117 by Sue Anne Hodges.

Bear illustration on page 35 by Harry S. Robins. Medicine Wheel on page 62 by Kim McLaughlin.

Printed in the United States of America

The Chakra System of Mount Desert Island is sponsored by the Society for the Study of Native Arts and Sciences, a nonprofit educational corporation whose goals are to develop an educational and crosscultural perspective linking various scientific, social, and artistic fields; to nurture a holistic view of arts, sciences, humanities, and healing; and to publish and distribute literature on the relationship of mind, body, and nature.

Library of Congress Cataloging-in-Publication Data

Kaiser, P. Chris.
    The chakra system of Mount Desert Island and its healing effects /
P. Chris. Kaiser
        p.   cm.
    ISBN 1-55643-271-2 (pbk.)
    1. Chakras—Miscellanea. 2. Mental healing. 3. Mount Desert
Island (Me.)—Miscellanea. 4. Mount Desert Island (Me.)—
Guidebooks. I. Title.
    BF1442.C53K35   1998
    917.41'45—dc21   98-19386
                                                        CIP

1   2   3   4   5   6   7   /   02   01   00   99   98

ACKNOWLEDGMENTS

I want to thank my wife, Karin, for her patience, her endless hours of editing, and her support, both psychological and financial, while I went about learning to embrace my tyrants.

I want to thank Gordon Longsworth at the Geographical Information Systems Library, College of the Atlantic in Bar Harbor, for spending hours with me in the creation of the maps for this book.

I want to thank Robin Farrin for the use of her camera and her darkroom.

I want to acknowledge the US Geological Survey for supplying the map of Mount Desert Island that appears on the cover of the book.

And I want to thank Richard Grossinger for coming back a second time.

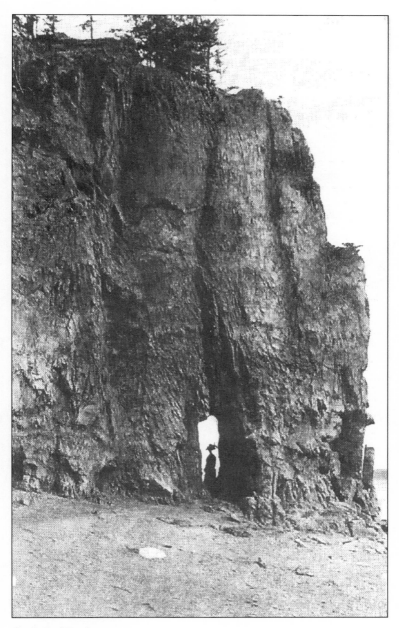

Cathedral Rock.

TABLE OF CONTENTS

PART I
THE CHAKRA SYSTEM OF MOUNT DESERT ISLAND

PART II
A BIRD'S-EYE-VIEW

PART III
THE SEVEN CHAKRAS ON CADILLAC MOUNTAIN

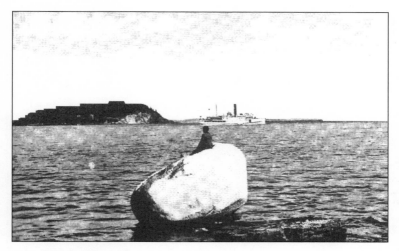

High tide at Balance Rock (circa 1862).

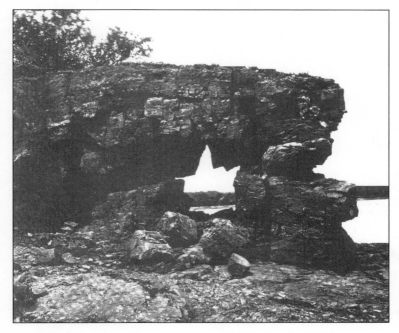

Star Crevice.

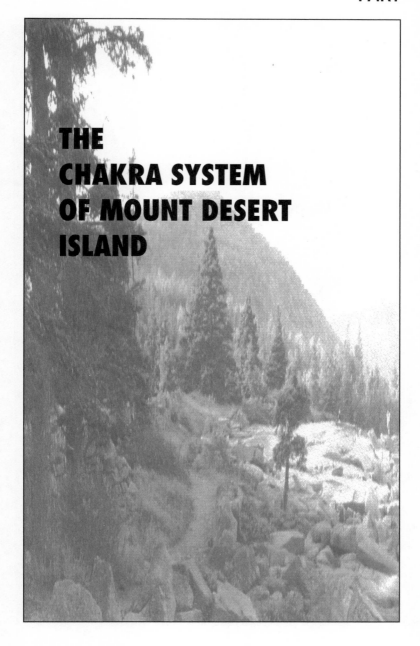

THE
CHAKRA SYSTEM
OF MOUNT DESERT
ISLAND

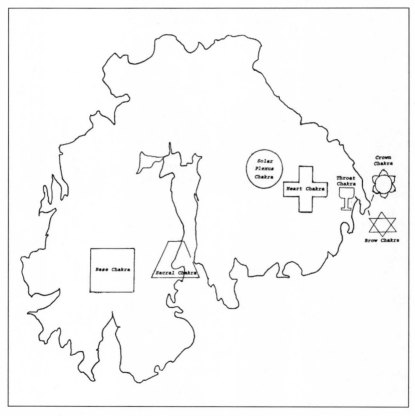

Figure 1: Chakra System Map, Mount Desert Island, Maine

CHAPTER 1

THE ISLAND OF
THE DESERT MOUNTAINS

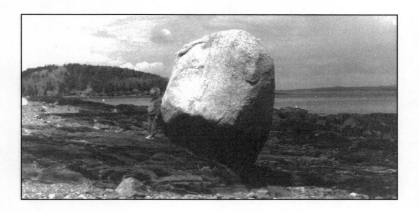

ON SEPTEMBER 5, 1604, the French explorer Samuel Champlain wrote in his journal, "The same day we passed also near an island about four or five leagues long . . . it is very high and notched in places so as to appear from the sea like a range of seven or eight mountains close together. The summits of most of them are bare of trees for they are nothing but rock . . . I named it the island of the desert mountains."

The island of "desert mountains" that Champlain saw is very much the same as what we see today, almost four hundred years later. But just as our lives involve numerous periods of

---

growth and change, this island has undergone many transformations, both physical and historic, both external and internal.

The northern coast of Maine originated about 500 million years ago as pressure and heat transformed a menu of sand, silt, and mud, transported from numerous rivers, combined with the sea's plant life to form the earliest bedrock of schist and gneiss. Known as the Ellsworth formation, this gruel produced mountains as lofty as the Rockies are today.

By comparison, we learn from Hesiod of a more poetically deified formation of the Earth, and the abodes of the gods, when he relates: "First of all, the Void came into being, next broad-bosomed Earth, the solid and eternal home of all, and Eros (Desire), the most beautiful of the immortal gods, who in every man and every god softens the sinews and overpowers the prudent purpose of the mind. Earth first produced starry Sky, equal in size with herself, to cover her on all sides. Next she produced the tall mountains, the pleasant haunts of the gods. . . ."

About 30 million years after the Ellsworth formation developed, another layer known as the Cranberry formation was laid down. The land once again sank into the sea, and new sediments collected, hardened, and emerged as a different bedrock of tuff (volcanic rock) and felsite. After they had accumulated to a height of several thousand feet, unrest and erosion set in. The unrest caused a folding of the volcanic layers, leaving many layers standing vertical before sinking a third time into the sea.

The sinking of the land into the sea is reminiscent of the destruction of Atlantis. June Chaplin of Bar Harbor was struck by the similarities between Plato's description of Atlantis and the history of Mount Desert Island and recently published a book entitled, *The Native Rock: The Geology of Acadia National Park*

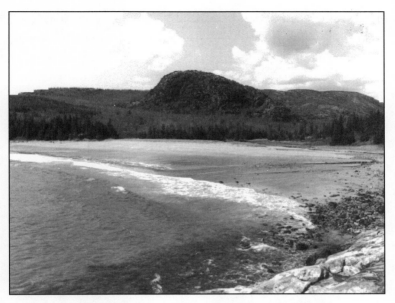

Sand Beach with the Beehive and Champlain Mountain behind it.

and Mount Desert Island, with Field Guide and Atlantis Comparison. In an interview with the *Bar Harbor Times* she states, "The island itself is almost exactly the same size [as Atlantis] and Somes Sound fits in well. The small central city described by Plato could have fit where the village of Somesville is now. Other evidence, including alleged similarities in Egyptian, Atlantan, and Native American pictographs, points to a Down East connection to the myth. Mount Desert Island also boasts the red, black, and white rocks described in the legend."

Next came what we call the Bar Harbor formation. Once again, rivers laden with rock and mud spilled their debris into the ocean. First gravel and stones accumulated; they were covered by hundreds of feet of sand and silt.

Transformed by heat and pressure, the gravel and stones fused into conglomerate; the silt formed predominantly brown, gray, and green siltstone.

After a long period of geological quiet, molten magma from deep in the Earth invaded the three formations on at least four relatively recent occasions. This first spewed diorite, next fine-grained granite, then coarse-grained granite, and finally a medium-grained granite.

It was the intrusion of the pink and green (the two colors of the heart chakra) coarse-grained granite that most dramatically altered the geological and spiritual architecture of the Mount Desert Island region. This layer was born far below the Earth's surface, consisting of a large plug of molasses-like magma, more than eight miles in diameter. As the plug pushed its way upwards, the roof of rocks over the plug collapsed into the magma. Here they were absorbed and then replaced by the new formation of coarse-grained granite that now defines most of the Mount Desert range.

Over many millennia the range appeared as a plain with an occasional low mountain, known as a monadnock, breaking its surface. Because of the flatness of the land, erosion occurred slowly, but eventually the land began to rise and tilt towards the sea, setting in motion rushing rivers that gouged steep valleys into the face of the range.

The final sculpting of the land that created what we know as Mount Desert Island happened as recently as 18,000 years ago when new glaciers spread across New England, their ice reaching thicknesses of almost two miles. Weighing ten to twelve million tons per acre, this flowing carpet flattened mountains and gouged new drainage systems. The major one on the island is Somes Sound, the only fiord on the whole east coast of North America.

As the glaciers migrated, they carried with them sand, stone, and boulders imbedded within their mass. These acted as gouging tools. They were often ultimately released great distances from their source, earning the largest boulders the name "erratics." The most conspicuous of these, known as Bubble Rock, sits to this day on South Bubble Mountain. Viewed from the Park Loop Road a little south of the auto road up Cadillac Mountain, it is precariously perched over a steep ravine just below the summit of the mountain.

About 15,000 years ago the ice mass reached the continental shelf, a hundred and fifty miles or so south of Mount Desert Island; it stopped growing and started to melt. As the margin of ice retreated, the land—which had been compressed approximately one foot for every three feet of ice upon it—rebounded, pushing back the inundating waters of the melting glacier. Finally, about 10,000 years ago, the current equilibrium between land and sea was reached. Present-day Acadia had been formed.

It was this land transformation that Champlain sailed into and called "Isle des Monts Deserts." But before that it was known by its former inhabitants, the Abnaki Indians, as Pemetic, "the sloping land." Preceding the Abnakis were two known prehistoric cultures. One, known as the Red Paint People because they painted their bodies with red and yellow ochre, dates back to 4000 B.C. The others were sometimes referred to as the "tuna fishermen" because tuna bones were found among their artifacts. Nobody seems to know how either tribe originated or what happened to them.

There is only conjecture concerning the first Europeans to encounter Mount Desert Island. Plutarch, about A.D. 75, in an imaginary dialogue with his antiquarian advisor, Sylla, raises the possibility of an oceanic crossing when Sylla shows an incredible familiarity with the lands to the west. He states, "Far o'er the brine an isle Ogygian lies distant from Britain five days' sail to the west. . . . those who come safely out of the perils of the sea land first on the outlying islands, which are inhabited by Greeks, and day after day, for thirty days, see the sun hidden for less than one hour. This is the night, with the darkness which is slight and of a twilight hue, and has a light over it from the west. [Greenland maybe?] There they spend ninety days . . . after which they pass on, now with help from the winds . . . to the great continent by which the Ocean is fringed is a voyage of about five thousand stades. . . ."

Another suggestion of migratory inhabitants from abroad lies in the megalithic ruins in North Salem, Massachusetts. Although their origin is still unknown, there is no hint of Christian influence. It's also believed that Irish monks preceded Columbus. Small caves dug into hillsides and lined with stones, believed to be meditation chambers, are attributed to their presence. Whether they built North Salem is questionable. Could it have been ancient Iberians? Around A.D. 1000 Leif Ericsson explored what is now the New England coast, staying one winter at a place he dubbed "Vinland," land of abundant grass, trees, and grapevines. Could this have been Mount Desert Island? Some people believe he is buried here and are still looking for his grave. Others postulate that fishermen from Portugal and Normandy arrived here. The earliest conventional historical records indicate that Steven Smith passed here around 1525 while searching for a strait leading to the Pacific.

There was little reference to Mount Desert Island over the next eighty years. Then Samuel Champlain, acting as pilot for Sieur de Monts, gave the island its present name. Sieur de Monts had a grant (from Henry IV, King of France)

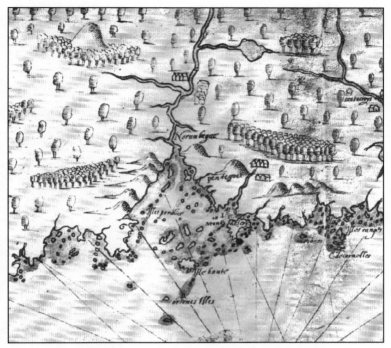

A section of Champlain's 1607 Chart of the Maine Coast, from the Kennebec River to Machias Bay.

to all the land in North America between what is now Philadelphia and Montreal. After setting up a trading post and colony on a small island in the St. Croix River along the present Maine-New Brunswick border, de Monts sent Champlain off to find Norumbega, a mythical city of wealth supposedly near present-day Bangor. It was on this exploratory trip that Champlain visited, mapped, and named Mount Desert Island, before continuing up the Penobscot River in search of Norumbega. Not finding any such city, he returned to St. Croix to report to de Monts his doubt concerning the city's existence. Although he probably sailed by Mount Desert Island again, that was his only actual visit.

Over the next one hundred fifty years the French and the English vied for control of the island and surrounding coast. They had differing views of how this should be attained. The English approach was to conquer and disperse the inhabitants, while the French urged friendship with the natives followed by religious conversion of them.

French Jesuit priests made the first settlement on Mount Desert Island nine years after Champlain's visit. Henry IV had been assassinated and Louis XIII had taken the throne. De Monts' grant was acquired by Antoinette de Pons, the Marquise de Guercheville, whose dream it was to establish a mission colony in the New World. With her backing, Father Pierre Biard and fifty-some passengers set sail on the *Jonas*, bound for Kadisquit (Abnaki for what is now Bangor). As the *Jonas* neared the Maine coast it was caught in thick fog and blown by gale winds into Frenchman Bay. Two days passed at anchor before the fog cleared and the Land of the Desert Mountains stood magnificently before them.

Thankful to have survived the journey, they rowed ashore near what is now Bar Harbor to hold mass and christen the land St. Sauveur. But as they pulled ashore, friendly Indians appeared, beseeching the newcomers to follow them to Fernald Point on Somes Sound, claiming that Chief Asticou, who was the head of the Penobscot branch of the Abnaki, was gravely ill and wanted to be baptized before dying. Unable to resist saving a soul, especially one of Asticou's standing, Biard and his group followed the Indians.

It turned out Asticou had only a cold. He had heard how friendly the French were and, wanting to have them settle near his summer residence, he had used this ruse to entice them. Seeing how beautiful Fernald Point was, with its ample fresh water, Biard decided to stay right there, so the first colony began.

No sooner had they started building their shelters and planting their crops than a British Captain, Samuel Argall, from the Virginia Colony at Jamestown (the same man who kidnapped Pocahontas), found their encampment. He had been ordered to demolish any and all French settlements between the Hudson and the St. Lawrence rivers and probably would have missed the Jesuit settlement tucked up Somes Sound if it hadn't been for some Indians who thought all Europeans were friendly. When the unknowing Indians told the English about their "brothers'" encampment, Argall bore down at once on the Jesuits, destroying the settlement and dispersing its inhabitants.

The English, however, neglected to settle on Mount Desert, probably because it was still too close to New France. Skirmishes between the English and the French continued over the possession of North America, but the island's greatest importance for Europeans over the next century and a half was as a prominent landmark for sailors, and a hiding place for French warships in Frenchman Bay.

In 1688 Antoine Laumet, who had immigrated to New France as a young man, ambitiously gave himself the title of Sieur Antoine de la Mothe Cadillac and obtained a grant from the Governor of Canada for a hundred thousand acres along the Maine coast, which included all of Mount Desert Island. For unknown reasons he and his bride spent only one summer on the island. He then departed for Montreal, entered the fur trade, and founded Detroit. His phony coat of arms still adorns the car of his name.

Finally in 1759, the British triumphed in Quebec, bringing an end to French domination of Maine and Canada. This also meant that the Indians, who had been allies to the French, had to leave their homes on the coast for more protected environs inland.

This left Mount Desert Island up for grabs for land speculators. Francis Bernard, Governor of Massachusetts (of which Maine was a part until 1820), laid a quick claim. He sought the island as compensation for personal expenses owed him by the colony.

Required by the terms of his deed to settle Mount Desert, Bernard instead found two men, Abraham Somes and James Richardson, eager to accept free land. They initiated the first permanent settlement on Mount Desert Island at the head of the sound; it was known as Somesville. Soon the American Revolution broke out, and Bernard lost his island anyway because of his loyalty to England.

After the war, two new claimants for the island came forth. One was Governor Bernard's son, Sir John Bernard, and the other was Sieur de la Mothe Cadillac's granddaughter, Marie Theresa de Gregoire. Sir John, unlike his father, had fought for the colonists, so he was awarded the western half of the island, and de Gregoire was given the eastern half. Neither claimant kept their holdings very long. Bernard immediately mortgaged his half and went back to England, while de Gregoire successively sold off parcels to support a meager living. She and her husband later died as paupers and were buried in Hulls Cove.

Over the next forty years Mount Desert Island flourished as roads and schools were built, and the land and its trees were cultivated. In 1844 Thomas Cole, a member of the Hudson

River School of American painting, enraptured by the island's beauty, began to paint scenes from Mount Desert and extol its virtues to his friends. Soon others came. Painters like Thomas Birch, William Hart, and Frederick Church, boarding with the locals, called themselves Rusticators.

As word of the island's beauty spread, Mount Desert became an international summer mecca for the wealthy. Hotels sprang up, and then stately mansions—euphemistically referred to as "cottages"—were built by such families as the Rockefellers, Carnegies, Fords, Vanderbilts, and Morgans. The stretch of shoreline between Bar Harbor and Salisbury Cove came to be known as "Millionaire's Row." Lavish parties ensued.

For four decades Mount Desert Island witnessed the comings and goings of the elite and wealthy. The Great Depression and World War II signaled the denouement of such extravagance. Then in 1947 the party ended as a massive fire raged through Millionaire's Row and much of the island for five days.

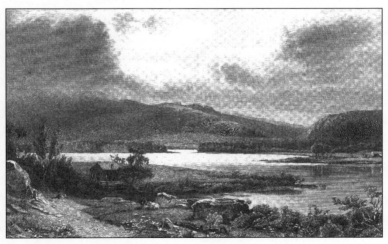

Somes Sound, as depicted in an 1861 engraving.

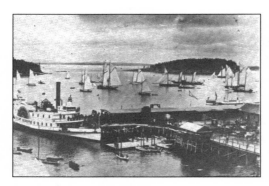

Bar Harbor pier, circa 1890.

Fed by eighty-mile-an-hour winds, it leveled forests and most of the great mansions in a matter of minutes, destroying more than 18,000 acres and 260 cottages.

Even though most of the mansions are gone, the Rusticators left an enduring landmark. Inspired by the philosophies of Emerson and Thoreau, they strove to protect the beauty that had drawn them here. One person especially, George B. Dorr, gave forty-three years of his time and energy, and most of his family wealth, to forming what is now Acadia National Park.

Dorr worked relentlessly acquiring land and fighting environmental political battles. Starting in 1901, he, Charles Eliot (the president of Harvard University), and ten others formed the Hancock County Trustees of Public Reservations, devoted to preserving places of interest for perpetual public use. On July 16, 1916, their efforts were rewarded when President Woodrow Wilson announced the formation of the 6000-acre Sieur de Monts National Monument. But Dorr wasn't satisfied. He wanted full National Park status. So, although sixty-three years of age, he labored and lobbied for three more years until President Wilson's approval was given on February 26, 1919, and Lafayette National Park was born.

Ten years later, land on Schoodic Peninsula was offered to the park, but the donors, being staunchly Anglophile, were reluctant to support a park with a French name. Realizing a park was a park no matter what the name, Dorr again petitioned Congress, and on January 19, 1929, Calvin Coolidge announced the establishment of Acadia National Park.

Another great patron of Acadia was John D. Rockefeller, Jr. Having both a philanthropic nature and a love for building roads and bridges, he conceived of a network of carriage paths that, accessing points of beauty in the park, would offer a quiet alterna-

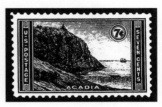

7¢ Stamp, showing woodcut of Great Head.

tive to the motor car. Today there are sixteen magnificent hand-cut stone bridges connected by fifty-seven miles of roads. A testament to Mr. Rockefeller's creativity and generosity, they meander through the island's hills and valleys seeking areas of solitude and natural splendor. Today, with four million people visiting the park every year, these roads are a haven for horses, bikers, and hikers.

Now the Island of Desert Mountains is on the verge of yet another transformation. This one is happening on an energetic level. Since transformation always occurs on an energetic level before it is seen in the physical, how and if it will affect the island's physical form, only time will tell. As you read about the chakra system of the island in the upcoming pages, you will have a better understanding of the energetics involved.

Many people see a reclining or sleeping woman in the silhouette of the island when viewed from the sea. I think it's appropriate to say that this woman is now waking up.

CHAPTER 2

THE EARTH EXPRESSES SYMBOLICALLY

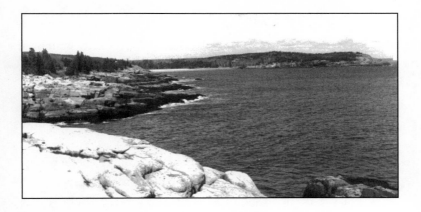

THIS BOOK IS ABOUT NOT ONLY the chakra system of Mount Desert Island but how to use these centers for healing and unifying the body/earth-mind-spirit continuum. Humankind is on the brink of an evolutionary leap in consciousness. We're learning to use the nine-tenths of our brain that has been dormant. You could say that we are on the threshold of a dream because we are venturing into, in a conscious way, two levels of consciousness that traditionally pertain to sleep—our dream state and our deep-sleep state.

According to science we have four levels of consciousness

The coastline along Ocean Drive.

that correspond to brainwave activity in cycles per second (cps). These four levels are beta, alpha, theta, and delta. Beta, 13–20 cps, is our waking state. Alpha, 10–12 cps, is our relaxed, meditative state. Theta, 5–9 cps, equates to our dream state. And delta, 0–4 cps, is our deep sleep state.

This is only one way of viewing these four levels. I learned from Tom Brown, Jr.,[1] that some indigenous peoples believe beta, which corresponds to the analytical mind, or left-brain activity, is a contrived state of mind. It doesn't truly exist. Also known as the island of reason, it was developed as a reference point for viewing the physical, which those ancient philosophers consider illusion. After all, thought, or spirit, which is energy, creates reality. Alpha is the doorway to the spiritual right brain, the primal mind, or island of silent knowledge. In theta you are one with spirit, and in delta you are spirit. In theta you also have complete control of the subconscious mind or low self.

If you compare the four levels to an iceberg, beta would correspond to the physical part that can be seen; alpha would represent the point of submersion into the water; theta would equate to the much larger base that supports the visible portion of the iceberg; and delta would be the ocean.

Historically, man has placed his focus on the analytical mind and the exploration of the physical world. In this period, referred to by the Hopi Indians as the World of Separation, the analytical mind is separate from the primal mind or spirit.

[1] Tom Brown, Jr., runs a wilderness survival school in northwestern New Jersey. Tom's mentor and teacher for ten years was Stalking Wolf, an Apache Elder who had been trained as a shaman and a scout. Tom has written numerous books about his tutelage under Stalking Wolf.

There is an imbalance between the will (male aspect) and the heart (female aspect). But now we are entering the World of Unity, which portends a balance of the left and right brains, our male and female sides, and the will and the heart. The heart is now being brought into the equation of every relationship. Therefore you are going to see an emphasis in this book on healing and strengthening the heart.

I believe the heart is the only key that opens all doors, the only chakra that can heal and unify the body/earth-mind-spirit continuum. It is the alpha, theta, and delta brainwaves; the connection to our low self, our high self, and all that is. The holistic mind sees the unity in all things, while the analytical mind sees things as separate. The heart is the chakra that so obviously exudes love for others, and for all life.

This shift into balance means learning a new set of rules. The left brain views the world literally but the right brain, resonating with our dream state, views the world symbolically. Time, which exists in the left brain, is absent in the right. The left brain obeys the laws of physics. The right brain (delta brainwave) transmutes the physical. The right brain is thereby the source of all miracles. In its domain we experience the oneness with all that is. With the left brain we look at the outer geography. With the right brain we experience the energetic behind the physical. In the left brain we communicate via language. In the right brain we communicate via feelings and images; the vehicle for communication is your imagination.

Exploring the theta brainwave means entering our subconscious mind or low self, and exploring the delta brainwave means ascending to our high self or the totality of ourselves. The middle self, by comparison, is the conscious part of ourselves. It equates to the beta brainwave and the analytical mind. It explores the island of reason. In order to access the "new" frontier of the primal mind, or the island of silent knowledge, we first need to get to know our low self. The key to this is our feelings. The low self is the seat of emotions and desires. It's the one that chokes up with tears at the movies, the one who wants the candy bar at the checkout line in the grocery store. The storehouse of all our knowledge, it runs the entire autonomic system of our bodies. Although it is not particularly analytical, it is very rational and habitual. It also communicates its feelings symbolically, which has some very interesting repercussions for our health, since the body is its primary medium of expression. It tends to take one's imposed belief system (which is often made up of many false beliefs), create habits out of them, and manifest these symbolically in one's body.

The two most important symbols to recognize when viewing the Earth, nature, and humans symbolically are the male and female aspects. We live in this duality, and its aspects are found not only in the physical world but also in our actions, our thoughts, and our feelings. The male aspect or yang energy is represented by an outward expression, while the feminine aspect or yin energy is represented by an inward expression. To send is yang; to receive is yin. To think is yang; to feel is yin. In humans, the left brain or analytical mind is yang and the right brain or feeling, intuitive mind is yin. Since the left brain runs the right side of the body and vice versa, the right side of the body represents the masculine arena and the left side of the body represents the feminine.

A good example of the low self expressing symbolically in our body is cardiovascular heart disease. The heart represents our feeling center. The expression of feelings, especially among males, is discouraged in today's society, and this fact has translated itself somatically into blocked arteries and heart attacks. A reflexology chart shows the microcosm of points on the bottom of the feet that corresponds to the organs of the body; all the organs are found on both feet except the heart, which is represented only on the left foot, the feminine. Interestingly, a heart attack is felt down the left (feminine/feeling) arm. *Chakra* is a Sanskrit word that means "spinning wheel," and it refers to energy vortices which look (to the psychically discerning eye) like tiny tornadoes attached to different parts of our body. The seven chakras are located at the base of the spine, the sacrum, the solar plexus, the heart, the throat, the brow, and the crown. They relate to survival (base), creativity and emotion (sacral area and low self), intellect and power (solar plexus and middle self), love (heart and high self), communication (throat), intuition (brow), and connection to spirit (crown). The chakras have both psychological and physiological functions. Their physical counterpart is the endocrine system and connected organs of the body. For instance, the sacral chakra interfuses the gonads and sexual organs and is also the seat of the low self, our center for feelings and creativity, as well as the origin of the two sexes, both inner and outer. The seven chakras vibrate to the seven colors of the rainbow and the seven notes of the musical scale. (See Figure 2.)

Besides being found on the body, chakras are also imbedded energetically and symbolically on the Earth in resonating macrocosmic and microcosmic forms. Like a hologram, each part of a chakra contains the whole. They appear sympathetically because the Earth and all of nature resonates at a theta brainwave. This is our dream state, and the language of dreams

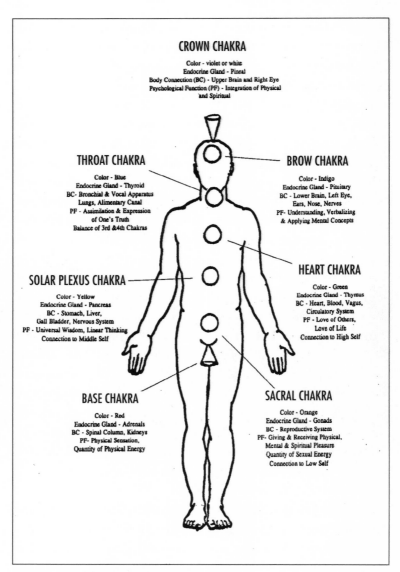

Figure 2: The Chakra System of the Human Body

is replicas and signatures. What you think of as a physical object, such as a rock or a tree, is also spirit constantly communicating symbolically. In this psychic geography the Hawaiian Islands are the heart chakra for the world, and Haleakala (House of the Sun) on Maui is the heart chakra for the Hawaiian Islands. Mount Desert Island plays a symbolic role in the passage of the sun through the Western Hemisphere because Cadillac Mountain is the first place in the United States touched by the morning sun. The heart is our connection to our high self, our spirit or god within. The word that best depicts spirit is light; the overwhelming replica of light on the physical plane is the sun.

The delta brainwave is our connection to our high self, the totality of ourselves. The high self is like a hand that has each of its fingers experiencing a different time-space continuum. To one finger, another finger may appear as a past or future life, which is a fallacy of the left brain's attempt to understand things sequentially. Actually, all lifetimes are happening at once and are constantly affecting each other. The delta brainwave, also known as the void, is the emptiness from which the present moment springs forth. It is the "NOW." Entering the World of Unity means unifying all of our lifetimes into now, the present. It means not only expanding our awareness to encompass all of our lifetimes, but embodying our high selves on the physical plane as Christ did.

Mount Desert Island has a lot of heart. Cadillac Mountain is an activator mountain (see Chapter 3). As the heart chakra on the island, it activates peoples' hearts. It, in turn, has seven chakras on its south ridge, the heart chakra of which is a pond in the shape of a heart. The island itself is in the shape of a human heart, so it magnifies feelings. Since your feelings are doorways to other dimensions, Mount Desert Island is a place for resolving alternate lifetimes, healing and opening your heart, and bringing it into balance with your will.

Especially now, I believe the heart is aiding us in making an evolutionary leap in consciousness. Presently we are transitioning out of the patriarchy, the use of the will without the heart, the analytical mind without the holistic mind. This leap in consciousness involves bringing the heart into balance with the will, and incorporating the nine-tenths of our brain we haven't been using. This primal mind, which equates to our feminine side (the heart), is made up of three levels of consciousness detected in brainwave activity as alpha, theta, and delta.

I hope the reader will understand that in viewing the island, it is important to remember that the universe forms in all dimensions simultaneously. The internal and external landscapes constantly impinge on each other. Power spots are links between realms of reality. Where Mount Desert lies in the physiographic realm corresponds to an area of great power in the astral-psychic realm. There are many such areas, including Sedona (Arizona), Stonehenge, Teotihuacan, Easter Island, certain caves in Australia, and so on. One can recognize the presence of the astral by there seeming to be something more in the landscape. The landscape has the prescience of more than three dimensions.

This book first describes the seven chakras on the island, then discusses the seven chakras on the south ridge of Cadillac Mountain. The most important thing when using this guide is to follow your heart and be conscious of your feelings. For this reason I've made the heart chakra, Cadillac Mountain, the next chapter in this book. An American Indian elder once said, "Every problem we solve with our head creates ten more problems, while those we solve with our heart stay solved." Although the chapters are arranged in a somewhat linear order, first up from the heart and then down, I urge you to go your own way. Look at the map of the chakra centers and see if you feel drawn to any particular one. I've included stories of healings at these different centers plus other anecdotes of interest in the hope that they act as springboards for your own journeys and healing experiences. From my heart to your heart, may love abide.

CHAPTER 3

THE HEART CHAKRA: CADILLAC MOUNTAIN

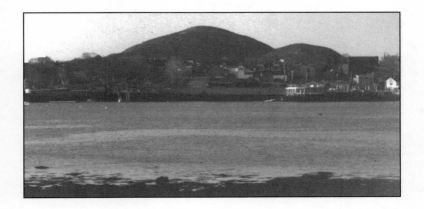

CADILLAC MOUNTAIN, as noted, is the heart chakra on Mount Desert Island. The heart is the only key that opens all doors, the doorway to our high self and the island of silent knowledge. Since Cadillac Mountain is the first place in the United States that is touched by the sun, it is a powerful place for accessing the spiritual part of ourselves.

Cadillac has hiking trails that ascend each of its four sides, coinciding with the four directions, much like a medicine wheel. There is also an auto road that goes to the top.

Bar Harbor as seen from Bar Island.

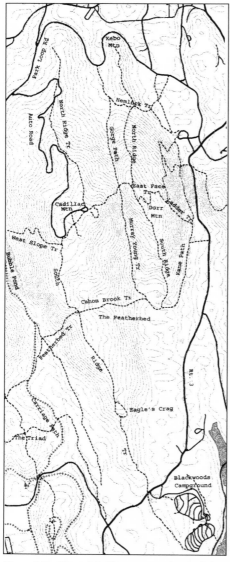

Figure 3. Trail Map of Cadillac Mountain/Heart Chakra

THE AUTO ROAD (very easy for cars, challenging for bikers) begins at the Park Loop Road, which can be accessed from a number of places. Those just coming onto the island may want to enter the park first at the Visitors Center off Route 3 just south of Hulls Cove. The Park Loop Road can be picked up at this point. Those in Bar Harbor can go west on Mount Desert Street, which becomes the Eagle Lake Road, or Route 233. Just outside of town, on the right, is another entrance onto the Loop Road. For those in the Northeast Harbor, Seal Harbor, Otter Creek, and Blackwoods Campground area, the

Loop Road can be accessed off Route 3 just across from the beach at Seal Harbor. In each case, signs can be followed to the mountain. There also is a fourth access point south of Bar Harbor just beyond the Jackson Lab, on the right side of Route 3. The Park Loop Road is one-way here, and it shortly becomes a toll road that takes you by the Seal Harbor park entrance.

THE NORTH RIDGE TRAIL (National Park Service rating: moderate; distance: 1.8 miles) is one of two trails going up the north side of Cadillac. The trailhead is marked by a cedar post on the right side of the Park Loop Road about four hundred yards after it becomes a one-way road. Parking is provided on the left side of the road. The closest access point is from Route 233. The trail starts out by climbing over large slabs of rock, then it levels out for a short while before ascending through the woods. After the woods, it bounds over more rocks, and then flirts with the auto road in a few places (scenic pullovers intrude). Here you can catch a breathtaking view of Bar Harbor below on the shore of Frenchman Bay. The small islands in the bay just off Bar Harbor are known as the Porcupine Islands because of their remarkable resemblance to that critter. At low tide you can see to the left of town the sand bar connecting Bar Island to Bar Harbor, giving the town its name. On the far side of the bay is Schoodic Peninsula. The tip of the peninsula is part of Acadia National Park.

The trail then dips away from the road and continues up over much exposed rock to the parking lot at the top. There you will find a gift shop and restrooms.

THE GORGE PATH (NPS rating: moderate; distance: 1.3 miles) is the other trail up the north side of Cadillac, although it actually lies in the valley between Cadillac and Dorr Mountains. The trailhead is on the right side of the Park Loop Road, about a half-mile beyond the North Ridge Trail. The trail follows Kebo Brook up into a gorge that is formed by the walls of these two mountains, which extend up thirty to forty feet. Near the top of the gorge you will encounter the East Face Trail to the left, which goes to the top of Dorr Mountain; the Murray Young Path straight ahead, which leads down the gorge on the other side of the notch; and the Notch Trail to the right, which goes to the top of Cadillac.

THE NOTCH TRAIL (NPS rating: strenuous; distance: .5 mile) is a short, steep footpath that runs from the Gorge Trail to the top of Cadillac.

THE WEST FACE TRAIL (NPS rating: strenuous; distance: 1.3 miles) is one of two paths going up the west side of Cadillac. It is the shortest and most direct route to the top of the mountain. From the parking area at Bubble Pond on the Park Loop Road, follow the path that leads towards the pond. At pond's edge continue left over a small footbridge to the base of the mountain. From here the trail climbs steadily to its intersection with the South Ridge Trail, a little south of the summit. The South Ridge Trail continues to wind over exposed pink and green granite, almost intersects the auto road near Blue Hill Overlook, then dips into a wooded valley before emerging at the top where a hotel stood prior to the 1947 fire. The gravel road to your left leads to the gift shop, restrooms, and a scenic walking path at the adjacent peak.

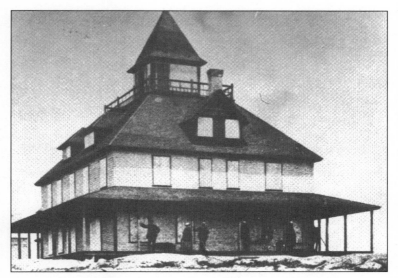

Located atop Cadillac Mountain, Green Mountain House was once a prominent landmark.

THE POND TRAIL (NPS rating: moderate; distance: 2.3 miles) is the other trail up the west side of Cadillac. It leads to the Featherbed, which is a pond in a valley on the south ridge of the mountain, about 1.2 miles south of the peak. This pond assumes the shape of a heart; it is the heart chakra on the mountain (see later chapters on the seven chakras on the south ridge of Cadillac). The Pond Trail can be accessed from the Park Loop Road at the south end of Jordan Pond, where there is a pull-off for parking. Except for the last .2 mile, which is very steep and strenuous, the trail offers a pleasant, easy stroll through mixed woods. The subsequent steep climb is worth it though, because it brings you onto some beautiful slabs of pink granite that are layered like huge steps. From here, the floor of the valley falls dramatically away to the west with Pemetic Mountain and the Triad rising beyond. Through the notch to the south is Seal Harbor looking out on the two Cranberry Islands (Great Cranberry is beyond Little Cranberry), with Sutton Island to the right and Baker Island to the left. The land mass across the water to the right is Manset, a part of Southwest Harbor. One hundred yards beyond the slabs of pink granite is the Featherbed.

THE CANON BROOK TRAIL (NPS rating: strenuous; distance: 1.5 miles) climbs the east face of Cadillac to the Featherbed. The trailhead is marked by a cedar post on the right side of Route 3 one-half mile south of the Tarn. There is a gravel pull-off on the right side of the road and a paved semi-circle on the left. The first half of this hike is quite moderate. It starts out through birch-dominated woods and crosses a beaver dam before intersecting with the Tarn Trail. Take a left here. The Tarn Trail remains flat for another .3 mile, then ascends abruptly to an intersection with the Dorr Mountain South Ridge Trail. Over the next .1 mile the trail descends to an intersection with the Canon Brook and the Murray Young Path. Follow the sign towards Eagle's Crag. The trail becomes steep and strenuous as it climbs for a half-mile alongside Canon Brook. About .4 mile up this ascent there is a friendly small pool, like a baptismal font, that you can sit in to the left of the brook. East on the medicine wheel correlates to new beginnings. A dip here can be very purifying and rejuvenating. Shortly after the pool, the trail steers away from the brook and allows you to catch your breath as it moderates over the next .3 mile to the Featherbed.

THE SOUTH RIDGE TRAIL (NPS rating: moderate; distance: 4.4 miles) spans the entire distance from Ocean Drive to the top of Cadillac, but most people just hike the 3.7 miles from Route 3. The trailhead here is marked by a cedar post and granite stairs on the west side of Route 3, just south of the entrance to Blackwoods Campground. The first mile of the trail is relatively flat and alternates between exposed roots, soft dirt, and rock. Then the trail starts rising more as it briefly ascends a boulder-strewn stream and passes a turnoff to Eagle's Crag, a .2-mile loop on the right. Just before passing the other end of the Eagle's Crag loop, the trail comes out of the woods and continues moderately to ascend over exposed rock with ever-increasing views of Champlain Mountain to the east, the Cranberry and Duck Islands to the south, and Pemetic Mountain with Blue Hill beyond in the distance to the west; until it dips to the Featherbed at 2.5 miles. From the Featherbed, the trail ascends steeply for .2 mile, then glides the next .8 mile over smooth rock with breathtaking views in all directions, including the Camden Hills 30 miles to the west, Mount Katahdin, Maine's highest peak, 75 miles to the north, and nearly all of the islands in Blue Hill and Frenchmen Bays. After this stretch, the trail dips into a wooded valley for .2 mile before arriving at the summit.

One day in February, nine months after moving to Mount Desert Island, I decided to climb the South Ridge Trail to the peak of Cadillac Mountain. I must have finished my gestation period on the island because this day was to become a real awakening, a turning point in my life.

It was a crystal clear day. The sun was almost blinding as it glistened and danced on the water. Snow on the ground was minimal, the temperature was in the twenties, and the wind was moderate. It was a perfect day for hiking.

As I mentally scanned the island upon first awakening, I felt an immediate pull in my gut to be on the South Ridge Trail of Cadillac. There was no hesitation, no second choice. Cadillac Mountain is part of a small range of mountains on Mount Desert Island that were ground down and rounded off eons ago when glaciers extended several hundred miles out into the Atlantic Ocean. Still, Cadillac is the tallest peak on the Eastern Seaboard and the highest headland north of Argentina. (Headland is measured by the distance between the height of the land and the depth of the sea.) The mountain is also considered to be a power spot and is sacred to the Penobscot Indians.

It felt so great to be out that I literally charged up the mountain, and it wasn't long before I reached a knoll which sits about three-fifths of the way up the ridge. Just north of the knoll the trail dips dramatically to a small glacial pond, or cirque, sitting in a depression known as the Featherbed. I walked to the center of the pond, which is all of thirty yards across, and the clarity of the sun bouncing off the ice was so warming and irresistible that I assumed a Tai Chi meditation stance and commenced to do a sun meditation. This involved placing my feet shoulder-width apart, bending my knees slightly, and tucking my pelvis forward so that my back was straight. Then I drew the sun in through my third eye and down to my heart, allowing it to expand and glow with feelings of warmth and love. I, in turn, sent these feelings in waves down through my body, while repeating a verbal meditation which is a take-off of the sun meditation found in the *Book of Runes* under the Rune Sowelu. It goes like this: "Oh great sun, the source of all power and light, whose rays illuminate the world, illuminate also this heart of mine, that I may become the clearest and purest channel of light possible within this lifetime."

For some reason my ability to feel my heart glow was great-ly enhanced that day. As I was getting lost in the joy of my own heart expanding, I was suddenly surprised by a gasp off to my right. Instantly I became aware of three or four people on either side of me. The reason for the gasp was a bear standing fifteen feet in front of us. Mind you now, both the people and the bear were an internal or shamanic experience, but nonetheless surprising. Even though I had been working shamanically with the bear, in all my previous journeys I had gone in search of him— never before had he spontaneously come to me. Since the people next to me seemed both excited and agi-tated, I suggested that they either hold their ground or retreat behind me. I then turned to the bear and asked if he had something he wished to tell me. By now, the bear and I were face to face; it was literally towering over me. It reminded me of my first encounter with the bear two and a half years before.

At that time, I was in the Never Summer Range on the western side of Rocky Mountain National Park in Colorado. I had been gradually opening my awareness to encompass communicating with plants and animals, and the prospect of connecting with a bear really engendered excitement in my being. I had been practicing for the encounter for quite a while, and affirming that my thoughts were creating my reality, I knew that as long as I persisted, sooner or later the bear would appear.

Every time I pictured the bear, it was like seeing an old friend. I imagined encountering him in the woods. He would not be aware of my presence until I suddenly came upon him, at which point he would gather himself up onto his hind legs to get a better look at me. I would stop and raise my right hand in a gesture of welcome. Then I would send out loving energy to him from my heart and connect it with his. At this point, he would noticeably relax, and still standing, he would raise a paw in an acknowledgement of friendship and respect. Then he would turn and amble off into the woods.

The encounter I actually had in Colorado was different in two respects. I was the one who was caught unaware, and the bear didn't appear very loving. Suddenly from out of nowhere the bear was in front of me. He was already standing and he was within ten feet of me. I stopped and tried to grip the ground through my sneakers with my toes, in case I had to flee. The bear, in turn, started towards me.

I felt that if I raised my arm in greeting it might agitate him, so I concentrated on connecting my heart with his. I knew it was my only hope. I knew we were all connected on the inner levels, and I used all the discipline I had to squelch my fear and radiate love to this 7-foot, 1700-pound potential friend. Still he came on. When he was directly in front and towering over me, I made a quick decision, because I felt I wasn't getting through to him. I knew that sometimes it took a blow to one's chakra in order to force it to open, so I gave the bear a sudden hard karate chop right in the center of his chest. Then I smiled at him and beamed all the love of which I was capable.

It worked. I felt the bear open and accept the love I was sending. His whole demeanor softened and he looked at me with knowingness, as if realizing who I was . . . his friend. Then I awoke from the vision.

Since then we have become good friends. In the encounter on Cadillac Mountain, I put a question to the bear. In response, he put his arms around me and gave me a hug filled with so much acceptance and contact that I actually broke down sobbing. I couldn't remember when anybody had accepted me so openly and totally. As I stood there releasing all emotion from my body, I in turn put my arms around the bear.

During this whole episode I was still cognizant of the outer world, thinking that if someone came over the trail and saw me standing on the frozen pond with my arms out in an embrace and sobbing, they would conclude I was nuts. Then I realized that at times like this when spirit is communicating, there would be no interruptions, so I allowed myself this final release.

I thanked the bear for coming and then turned to continue up the mountain. At this point I was so totally relaxed, in the moment, and devoid of expectation that it didn't matter to me where I went or when I got there. The heart chakra was doing its thing. It was pure joy to be walking on the mountain, feeling its energy and allowing myself to be drawn to whatever caught my attention. The primal energy of the mountain flowed through my body and felt so good I couldn't get enough of it. I felt literally weightless.

As I neared the top I noticed a large sign along the road that wound up the mountain. Curious to see where I was, I headed in its direction. As I stepped onto the road I suddenly felt twenty pounds heavier. Tired, my guts queasy, I wanted to sit down and rest. Just seconds before I had felt so weightless and energized that I couldn't figure out why this was happening. Then I realized—the pavement was actually blocking the energy of the mountain from coming through. The mountain's energy was so palpable yet so radiatingly subtle. But the road was like being on a dead substance. I began to realize how towns and cities, and even our houses, affect the way we feel. My first response, other than getting off the road, was indignation at the intrusion of this dead substance on the mountain. Soon, though, I was to learn of its higher purpose.

I continued on, and as I reached the top I headed for what appeared to be the highest point, a large rock. As I climbed up onto it, I spontaneously called out, "Oh great spirit of the mountain, I have come as a voice to pass on your wisdom to the people. Is there anything you wish me to convey?" I felt a soothing, healing, loving vibration run up my legs, through my body, and out my head. As it got stronger it felt as if my belly were expanding into a round ball. I imagined the Earth as she was giving birth to a new form.

I knew beyond a doubt that the Earth is a live sentient being, evolving just as we are. Cadillac had brought me to the threshold of a new and higher vibration. I understood, in resonance with the Earth, that we as a planet are going from a seven-chakra system to a twelve-chakra system. This seemed to correlate with the Earth's energy body evolving geometrically to a pentadodecahedron, which is twelve stars joined together with their pentacles touching. Joel Jochman, the author of *Rolling Thunder: The Coming Earth Changes*, believes that such a prophecy occurs symbolically in the Bible as the new Jerusalem, a city as high as it is wide and deep. The twelve stars represent the twelve gates.

The vision on Cadillac also communicated to me that many indigenous peoples were and are aware of the Earth's and humanity's leap in evolution. The Hopis, for instance, describe our coming transition from the Fourth World of separation (the patriarchy) into the Fifth World of unity (a balance of the male and female). Their elders say that between each world the Earth has geologically and psychospiritually changed. The last changes were by water (referred to in the Bible as the Great Flood); the coming changes are to be by both water and fire. This Hopi transition also correlates with the end of the Mayan calendar in 2012.

I suspected these changes were beginning to take place, but now I was being shown what the Earth felt. I could feel the Earth stretching and growing and expanding. As I stood there, sobs again racked my body. I felt the love that welled up inside her core, building, pushing out. The feeling of love had started deep in her center and was working its way out; the inside of my belly felt so warm and glowing that I didn't know how to contain the joy I was feeling. A broadcast emanated from the Cadillac chakra. The Earth wanted to stretch, inhale deeply, and expand. Areas of potential violence or low vibration around the world felt taut and inflexible on my skin, as though it would rip apart cataclysmically as the pressure mounted.

I floated home and tried to convey to some of my friends what happened. Words seemed so inadequate. I went to bed early that night wondering if I had really experienced what I had. I was awakened by a voice in my head repeating, "I am the Mountain," over and over. I looked at my watch; it was 3 AM. I wanted to sleep, but the voice was so insistent that I grabbed paper and pencil and started recording.

The information initially came three or four words at a time; then it shifted to sentences, to paragraphs, and finally chapters. It was like looking through a camera as the lens shifted from narrow to wide angle. By 6 AM I had read a whole book's worth of information. It was frustrating not being able to write everything down, but the information came so fast that all I could do was transcribe chapter headings. It wasn't long before I mentally crashed and fell asleep again.

The next morning I was awakened at 5 AM, and I thanked the Mountain for being a little more considerate. The process of transmission continued off and on over the next several weeks. The following is what I received from my new teacher:

I am the Mountain. I come to speak to you of many changes that will be taking place. As I stretch and grow, the aspects of myself that are here today will no longer be viable in the future. What I mean is that I will no longer be the same. I am alive and I am growing into a being that is far greater than what I am now.

I have been here for eons of time and have experienced many things, the coming and going of many eras. I have sat under ice and been exposed to the elements. Now it is time to tell people of my purpose upon the Earth.

You think only you have purpose; I am here to help the Earth in her growth process. Just as the heart is part of the human body and helps sustain it, it is a separate organ and entity in and of itself. Actually, it is a gateway to higher energies, with the ability to metabolize feelings. So it is with me. I am a part of the Earth and I perform a very definite function; yet I am a self-contained entity, feeling, growing, learning. I am part of and one with the Earth, the all that is; yet I am the Mountain. So it is with you.

As you walk on me you blend with my energies, my knowing. You come away with knowledge that you are not often consciously aware of. You have built a road on me and you come to me by the millions to learn of my knowledge—knowledge that is passed onto you on the cellular level.

You are being awakened. You don't know why you come, but you come to me. I am an activation point. I am activating the Earth and I am activating you. After you walk on me changes start to take place in your life. Little did you know, it was my energy that triggered the change. You needed to bathe yourself in my energy field to activate your change and that is why you came. But it is a two-way street. I am an acupuncture point on the Earth. I activate change within the Earth and within you, but I also need you to activate me.

There are people arriving here now on the island who will be working with me and through me to activate the energies of the Earth just as their brothers, the Native Americans, did before them. There are those who can feel the energy vibration that I send out. Remember, all is energy. Each and every thing that you perceive is a vibration. Everything has its own vibration, and information is encoded within each vibration, which you perceive as form and knowledge.

As I am activated, in turn the Earth will be activated. My vibratory rate will not only become stronger, but it will be raised to a higher octave. I am one of many activation points on the Earth.

I am the Mountain. I come to pass on the knowledge of the ages. For me it has been just a short time, for you it appears as eons. There were times when I could look out over the valley and see lush green grass blowing in the wind, and there were times when all was black and charred with the ash of fire. I have sat and pondered myself while blanketed in ice, and I have stood as a beacon to be seen miles out at sea on a clear day.

To you I am a mound of earth to be climbed and walked over. Little do you realize that I have life and awareness. I am able to keep track of everything that happens upon me. I am a historical record not only of myself but of all that is in my view. Being one with all, I know and am all things. I will speak to you if you will just approach me in reverence and be open in your heart and your mind to what I have to say.

Many have walked upon me and felt my song. They have come away changed, often not realizing the effect I have had upon them. I have been whispering to all of you to hear what is being said in your hearts.

I am the heart. I magnify that which you are feeling. If your heart is closed and angry, I will make you feel that in your whole being until you can recognize it in yourself and change. Either that or you will die from your pain.

Presently my energy is contained or else you would not be able to come near me. You could not approach me safely unless you were clear of all negative thoughts and feelings. Otherwise the anger that you brought with you would explode within you and drive you over the edge with terror.

I am the heart. I activate. I am pure. I cannot be tamed. The energy that I exude now, the vibration at which I resonate, is going to become stronger. Those who walk on me now and feel my joy will throw their arms out from their chests in an attempt to fill themselves further with my bliss. Those who block this joy with their negative feelings will crumble to the ground, constricted with the agony of what they hold cooped up within themselves.

Time is running out on the sustainers of negative thought patterns. Acceleration is going on in the many spheres; your thoughts are creating your own reality faster, ever faster. The universe is aiding you in being able to see what you are sending out. Thoughts on war will bring war into your life and take everything you hold precious. If you still can't let go, then it will take you. If you are following your heart and your thoughts are in harmony, then you will ride the waves of your bliss to heights you never dreamed possible. ¡

¡I am the Mountain. I am here to bring you the news of a fresh way of seeing the world. First it is happening on a vibrational level; soon you will see it on a physical level.

I am bringing news of a new order. There is no separation. Everyone will realize this. You think that you are alone in your journey, but in truth we are all connected on the inner levels. A time is coming when this knowledge will be accepted once again, and the way that you see the world and each other will change.

I am here to wake you up. Come out of your dream, yon illusion, and observe the world as it is. You are dreamer and you are dreamed.

I am the Mountain and I speak to you of many changes to come. You are being told that I was formed by certain geological conditions. This is all true but it is only a small part of the picture. I am first an expression of energy, and even before that an intent of thought. I am a representation of what you are. Just as the intent of thought created me, your intent is creating what you see before you.

We are equals, you and I. We come from the same source and are not dissimilar in our makeup. I contain elements of the Earth and so do you. I have a communications network of quartz crystals; you also are crystalline beings.

You think I am incapable of thought and interactions. You have forgotten how we interact. You have forsaken listening inward for the glitter of the outer world. You have forgotten that the outer world is but a reflection of the inner world. The inner world creates the outer world, but the outer world is only a fraction of the inner world. So it is with me. What you see is only a fraction of what I am. You look at me and see only a mountain.

Be open and receptive and I will fill you with my wisdom, for I have been here a long time. Wake up and become aware. You are capable of so much more. If you fail to listen you will be missing the opportunity of many lifetimes. Actually, you are here now to take advantage of this opportunity. You chose to be here.

CHAPTER 4

THE THROAT, BROW, AND CROWN CHAKRAS: SAND BEACH AND GREAT HEAD

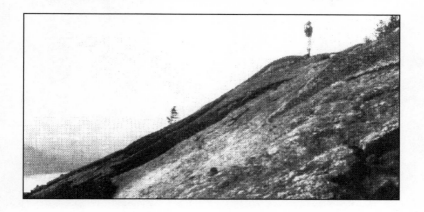

SAND BEACH REPRESENTS the throat chakra, and Great Head represents the brow and crown chakras. The throat chakra is the chakra of expression. The male aspect of this chakra activates speaking things into being, while the feminine aspect equates to listening and taking responsibility for our actions. In its purest sense, I believe the throat or fifth chakra equates to the Hopi Fifth World of unity, which is a balance of the third and fourth chakras, or the will and the heart.

The brow chakra, located at the third eye (between the eyebrows), is the node of intuition. In its purest sense, it sees

The cliffs of Green Mountain.

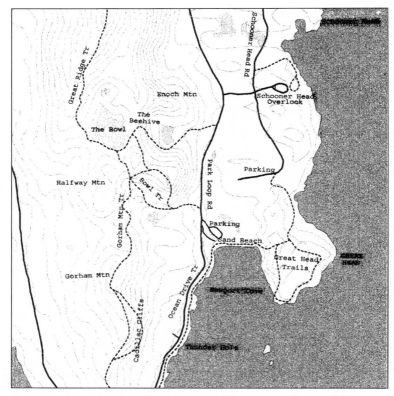

Figure 4: Trail Map of Sand Beach and Great Head / Throat, Brow, and Crown Chakras

all life forms as manifestations of God. Its earthly, feminine function grasps mental concepts, while its masculine counterpart carries out ideas practically.

The crown chakra is our connection to our higher mind, our knowingness. It pertains to the integration of our physical and spiritual makeup, i.e., the body-mind-spirit continuum. You can visit these in the macrocosm.

To get to Sand Beach, take the Park Loop Road from either the Visitors Center on Route 3 just south of Hulls Cove; or, from Route 233 just west of Bar Harbor, head towards Cadillac Mountain. Just before reaching Cadillac, turn left onto the one-way section of the Loop Road, and follow it to the toll booth. Sand Beach parking area is on the left about two hundred yards beyond the toll booth.

If you wish to avoid the toll, plus Ocean Drive and Thunder Hole, you can take a left just before the toll booth towards Schooner Head, and then the next right onto Schooner Head Road. There is a small parking lot that fills up quickly about a mile down the road. At the edge of the parking lot is a dirt path. A stone's throw beyond is a cedar post at the junction of two paths. The path to the left leads to Great Head. The path straight ahead goes to Sand Beach, a gentle quarter-mile walk. At a second junction in the trail to Sand Beach, take either fork.

THE GREAT HEAD TRAIL (NPS rating: moderate; distance: 1.3 miles). To get to Great Head from Sand Beach, walk the length of the beach to the end opposite the parking area. Here you will see an old cedar post and some granite stairs going up the hillside. At the top, the trail to the left will take you to the parking area on Schooner Head Road. Take the unmarked path to the right. Within one hundred yards you will see blue trail markers that lead up over the rocks to the tip of the peninsula.

An alternate trail to the tip of the peninsula hugs the edge of the shore, sometimes twenty to thirty feet above the water; it can be found about one hundred yards to the right of the granite steps. A large slab of rock at the water's edge forms the embankment. At the top of the slab you will see a well-worn path.

After rounding the point of the peninsula, the path veers away from the water and gradually ascends to the head's highest point, 145 feet above the sea. The ruins that you see here were once a tea house, built around 1915. From here the trail descends into a birch grove along an often soggy path. The first cedar post marks a trail that leads directly up over the ridge to the left, offering fine views of Gorham Mountain, the Beehive, the Precipice on Champlain, and the south ridge of Cadillac. Then the trail drops back to the granite stairs where you started, making a loop of 1.3 miles. The second cedar post is the one by the Schooner Head parking area. Go left here and follow the path for .3 mile to Sand Beach.

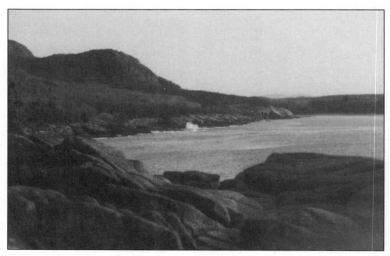

Great Head, the highest headland on the East Coast.

I first visited Sand Beach and walked the Great Head loop back in the late sixties when I was going to school in Maine. Little did I know then that I would return almost thirty years later. Now when people ask me what brought me here, I tell them that I had an appointment with an island and a mountain. I do feel that I have been guided here to remember my connection with the Earth, and to help others remember. In one sense the process of remembering has been analogous to unfolding wings that have been dormant for decades, and learning anew to fly. Yet in another sense it has been similar to putting together an intricate puzzle, the pieces of which are represented by people, places, and events, some of which follow. Learning about the throat chakra on Mount Desert Island was one of those intricate puzzles, a major piece of which came from an East Indian teacher, Gurumayi.

Before coming to Mount Desert Island I lived in New Harbor, Maine, for two years. While there I became friends with a group practicing Siddha yoga. The organization is head-quartered in Ganeshpuri, India, and is presently headed by a woman named Gurumayi Chidvilasananda.

One day prior to my moving to Mount Desert Island, my friend Gail called and asked if I could come over that evening. She and her husband had just finished the construction of a fireplace in a room on the end of their house, and that evening, with the lighting of a fire in the new fireplace, they were dedicating the room as an informal Siddha yoga center.

Shortly after I arrived the ceremony began. As we gathered around the growing fire, I distinctly felt someone staring at my back. I turned around and found myself staring into Gurumayi's eyes, particularly her dominant left eye. (The left

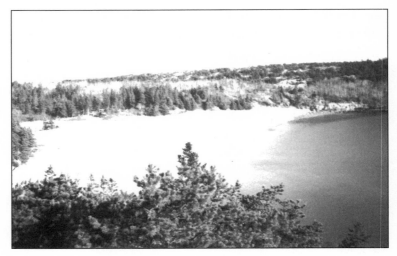

Sand Beach with a portion of Great Head in the distance.

eye accesses the right brain, which is the feminine, feeling side of our being.) Actually it was a framed poster of her hanging on the wall, a small altar underneath. As I stared in astonishment, her facial features suddenly changed. I assumed it was my imagination, but when I looked back she did it again. I could barely contain myself at this point. It was all I could do to wait in place until the fire ceremony was completed. I maneuvered behind Gail and huddled there with my hands up, ready to shake her shoulders the moment she was finished.

Fortunately it was a short ceremony. As Gail turned I started blubbering, stuttering, and pointing to Gurumayi. I wanted Gail to share my excitement, but she just looked at me calmly and assured me that Gurumayi was entirely capable of such things. To make a long story short, I concluded that Gurumayi helps take people into their right brain, back to the union and oneness of the heart. When we are able to let go of left-brain dominance, we see much more—not only in the physical plane, but beyond the physical.

One day after moving to Mount Desert Island, I was pondering this interconnectedness and attempting to view the island symbolically. It dawned on me that Great Head represents the island's symbolic expression of the brow and crown chakras, which made Sand Beach the throat chakra.

I have always considered Sand Beach a healing place and have gone there to be restored whenever I feel tired and run down. I also consider it special because it's not really made of sand; it looks like sand but is actually crushed shells. The number of shells it would take to make such a beach, and the energy and intention needed to bring them all to that one spot are not unlike the energy and intention it would take to collect the stars in a galaxy. Being the throat chakra, Sand Beach carries the vibration of the Fifth World of unity. Energetically it represents a balance of the will and the heart. I recommend a visit there when inner or cosmic balance is your goal. Let your presence merge with the energy beyond time and space that has made the beach.

CHAPTER 5

THE SOLAR PLEXUS CHAKRA: EAGLE LAKE

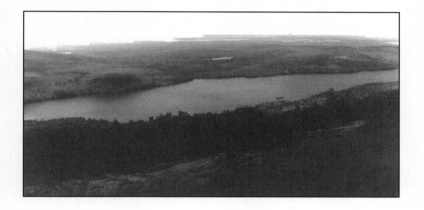

THE SOLAR PLEXUS CHAKRA embodies the male aspect—linear thinking and the use of the will. Also the home of the middle self, this chakra pertains to self-image, one's intention of who he or she is within the universe.

I often use the term "stalker" to describe a person who is focused on their solar plexus chakra, or their will. In the purest sense, a stalker is one who is adept at exploring the outer world, or the physical. In patriarchal cultures, however, a stalker lacks a balance between the will and the heart and is someone who uses power and intellect to control others. Every

---

Eagle Lake as seen from the top of Cadillac Mountain.

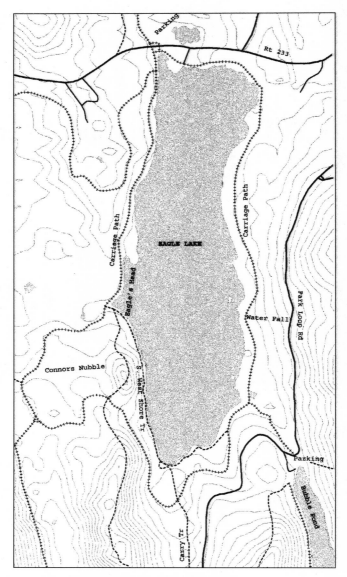

Figure 5: Trail Map of Eagle Lake / Solar Plexus Chakra

relationship, whether it be friendship, marriage, business, politics or whatever, contains a stalker and a dreamer, a will person and a heart person. A "heart person" needs to learn to strengthen his or her will, or to stand strong in the heart, whereas a "will person" needs to learn to open his or her heart because power is nothing without compassion. Being conscious of the ramifications of this equation in our daily lives can greatly facilitate achieving balance.

The solar plexus chakra on Mount Desert Island is located at Eagle Lake, just off Eagle Lake Road. From the head of the island take Route 102 south where it branches off Route 3 (at the Parkadia Exxon), and follow it to the stoplight in Somesville. Turn left onto Route 198, go about one mile, and turn left again onto Route 233. This is Eagle Lake Road. There is a parking area at the north end of the lake on Route 233, and another one on the Park Loop Road at Bubble Pond. To get to the Bubble Pond parking area, continue past Eagle Lake on Route 233, go up a long hill, under an overpass, and then take an immediate left onto the Park Loop Road. From here take your first left, then bear right until you see signs for the pond.

To get to Eagle Lake from Bar Harbor simply follow Mount Desert Street (which is Route 233) west out of town until you reach Eagle Lake.

Eagle Lake is surrounded by a six-mile carriage path ideal for biking, hiking, and (in the winter) cross-country skiing. On the southwest side of the lake there is also a short hiking trail (the Eagle Lake Shore Trail), which provides great views of the lake.

THE EAGLE LAKE SHORE TRAIL (NPS rating: moderate; distance: 1.6 miles) is best located from the parking area at Bubble Pond. Once at the parking area, cross the park road and take the carriage path to where it intersects the path around Eagle Lake. Turn left here and continue a short way until you see a sign-post on your right marking the Shore Trail. From the Shore Trail you can access Connors Nubble, which rises to the west above the lake. As you enter the Shore Path, go left. A sign-post marks an intersection with the Carry Trail, an old Indian path that once connected Eagle Lake with Jordan Pond. Continuing on, you will see the vertical sides of the Nubble appear. A sign marks the trail up over Connors Nubble. The top of Connors Nubble affords expansive views of Eagle Lake as well as Cadillac, Pemetic, North and South Bubbles, Penobscot, and Sargent Mountains.

To go back to the parking area, continue on the path away from the lake until you reach the carriage path that circles it.

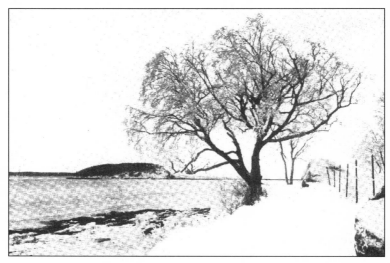

The shore path in winter.

Take a left onto the carriage path and retrace your steps back past where you entered the Eagle Lake Shore Trail to the carriage path on your right that leads back to your car.

Another point of interest here is a stream on the east side of the lake that flows from Cadillac Mountain into Eagle Lake. A small wooden bridge along the carriage path that surrounds the lake goes over the stream. Located about two-thirds of the way between the entrance to the carriage path at the Eagle Lake parking area (going left) and the intersection where you would turn left to go to the Bubble Lake parking area, the stream sometimes dries up, but when it is running, it forms a small waterfall a stone's throw upstream from the bridge. I have found this to be an ideal place for meditating and reprogramming dysfunctional habits stored in the subconscious mind. The negative ions thrown off by the running water are beneficial, but more important is the symbolic gesture expressed by the Earth at this location. Water manifests the feminine aspect, and here the heart (Cadillac Mountain) is being brought to the will (Eagle Lake), a very effective aid to the task we face of balancing our will with our heart.

An exercise that you may want to practice here is the "breath to heart" technique. I learned this also from Tom Brown, Jr. Tom teaches this technique as part of a Tracking and Awareness course. Part of his course involves becoming aware of the energetic connection between nature and humankind, which means changing one's consciousness from the analytical to the primal mind by slowing down the heart. You will notice that when you hold your breath, or when you exhale after holding your breath, you can feel your heart beating. As you experience the thump, concentrate on it and

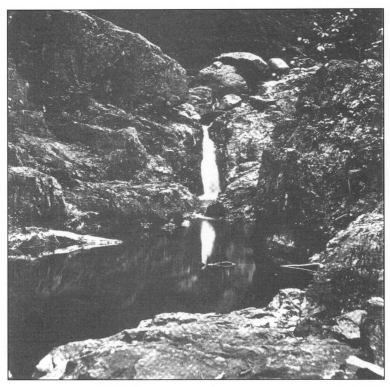

Duck Brook, the outlet for Eagle Lake.

consciously direct it to slow down. Keep at it; as the heart slows, so also does the mind.

Another technique Tom teaches for entering the primal mind combines wide-angle vision with a "fox walk." Wide-angle vision concentrates on the entire range of vision, both front and peripheral. The "fox walk" is a technique for walking silently in the woods. To perform it, keep your weight on one leg and use your other leg as a feeler. Place the outside of the ball of the foot of your feeler leg softly to the ground. Then gently roll the rest of the ball of the foot onto the ground. Finally, as the heel is quietly brought down, your weight is gradually shifted to that foot. Be careful the whole time to maintain silence. When you combine the "fox walk" with wide-angle vision, the fusion of the two acts to "stop the world" (to borrow a phrase from Carlos Castaneda). It brings you, with a slam, into the moment—no time, the primal mind.

A third technique for entering the primal mind is to spend four days on the Earth away from civilization. The Earth resonates at 7.8 cycles per second, which equates to a good solid theta brainwave. At theta you become one with spirit, attuned to the energy vibrations of nature, animals, and humans. You also gain complete command of the low self. I had this experience at Tom's school the day he taught us the "breath to heart" technique combined with being on the Earth (dwelling in the wilderness) for four days. It was a difficult period in my life, for I had recently separated from my wife and family.

Tom waited until we had been out of civilization for the requisite four days. He then reviewed the "breath to heart" technique. First he led us in some relaxation exercises. We spent time tensing the different muscle groups of our body for several seconds and then relaxing them. After that we tensed our full body and then relaxed it. Then Tom guided us through a hypnotic visualization that left us melting into the Earth. After doing the "breath to heart," we were told to scan the interior of our bodies from head to foot. If we encountered any pain or discomfort, we were to go into it and command it to leave. By venturing into the primal mind, we become attuned to the energetic world that supports the physical. The Chinese and Japanese have been exploring this realm for centuries via such disciplines as Tai Chi, Chi Kung, and Reiki.

As I scanned my body I suddenly became aware of a burning pain in my left testicle. I also realized that it had been going on for a while unfelt and eclipsed by the overwhelming guilt I was feeling over having left my family. As I attempted to enter the pain, I was surprised at the ease with which I was able to move into its center. I was even more surprised when it suddenly stopped at my command. Not only did it stop; it never returned.

Tom was trying to teach us to have this same commanding oneness with nature. The Pine Barrens of New Jersey are infested with ticks, and each night before crawling into our sleeping bags we would have to detick ourselves, often with the help of another person. My routine after deticking was to crawl into my bag, lie perfectly still, and wait to see if any ticks would start moving. If I felt any moving, I would get them.

That night, after magically stopping the pain in my left testicle, I did the deticking ritual and crawled into my bag. It had been a rewarding day, filled with new information and new accomplishments, but now I just wanted to be alone so I could mull over all that happened. As I lay quietly in my bed I suddenly felt a movement. I couldn't believe what was happening. I tore open my sleeping bag, grabbed my flashlight, and ripped down my underwear for verification. There on my left testicle was a tick, firmly imbedded.

I had been taught that when a tick is imbedded, you need to touch a match to it so it will back out and not leave its head in your skin. But I was so disgusted that I grabbed tick and skin and hair, and yanked. After annihilating the tick in my frenzy to rid myself of it, I went back to assess the damage. I noticed a pea-size growth in my testicle. Intuitively I knew that my intense feelings of guilt over leaving my family had embodied there. I also knew that I had put a stop to the growth earlier that day. As I pondered the interesting points of "coincidence" among the pain, the tick, and my newfound knowledge, I began to see that my higher self had incorporated all these aspects into one fascinating lesson in order to advance my knowledge into knowing.

I gave thanks to the spirit of the tick that I had just annihilated for playing its role so well. I now knew that it was just cooperating with the grand scheme in order to get my attention where it needed to be. I started using Reiki (Japanese healing technique for channeling universal life force) on myself daily, and within a month the growth disintegrated and disappeared.

Vision quest is another worthwhile practice for utilizing the energy centers on Mount Desert Island. This enables one to leave the physical geography and travel inward to the astral corridors and the spirit forms that dwell there. A vision quest usually entails going out on the land, away from civilization, for a number of days (ideally four or more), and fasting while seeking a vision or supernatural guidance. A circle may be drawn on the ground. This is your home for the duration of the quest. You must stay within.

It was during a vision quest on the west side of Cadillac that I became aware that Eagle Lake was the geographical manifestation of the third chakra. I also became aware that this was my last lifetime in the World of Separation before the World of Unity. Since all of our lifetimes in the World of Separation are being unified, NOW is the time to resolve anything that has been left unresolved. During this quest of four days, I fasted with only water. This ritual allowed me to resolve a number of my current issues as well as those of an alternate lifetime of enslavement that had been physically plaguing me.

Cadillac Mountain is a medicine wheel, a symbolic representation of the universe. The Native American medicine wheel, among many other things, contains the four directions coinciding with the four periods of the day, the four seasons, the four elements, and the four races. A tool for movement and change, the four directions of the wheel also represent four aspects of transformation: north—wisdom, east—illumination, south—growth, and west—introspection. The plant, animal, and mineral kingdoms are also represented in the wheel, and each direction has a spirit keeper and an animal totem. Realizing that we are one with all the elements of the wheel, and that they are therefore inside us, allows us to enter the wheel, hence ourselves, to find any answers we need.

The west side of Cadillac, symbolic of introspection and the end of the day, is also the direction of the shaman's death in vision quest, or the death of the ego. I wanted to culminate some stalker lessons in my life, some third-chakra stuff. Questing on the west side of Cadillac, which overlooks Eagle Lake, was more than symbolic to me—it felt like a birthright. I had gone to the mountain in utmost humility and asked for wisdom, and the mountain had spoken to me. I simply wanted to sit and fast and commune with the mountain once again.

(Please understand that the National Park Service prohibits back-country camping in Acadia. Perhaps some day they will set aside areas or give special permits, but in the meantime, one can achieve tremendous healing with daily visits.)

On the third morning of my quest I awoke knowing that I needed to cleanse my chakras. When journeying in the primal mind, imagination and intent become the vehicles for movement and communication. You stop each chakra and with the aid of your psychic or third eye and your imagination, clean out any debris you find with either your physical or your psychic hand. Afterwards you move your hand in a circular clockwise fashion over the chakra while envisioning it starting to spin.

I was sitting inside a triangle formed by three cedar trees. They were my companions and my shelter from prying eyes. About fifteen feet in front of me and a little to my left were the remains of an old tree standing about six feet high. The previous afternoon a woodpecker had landed on the tree, looked at me, then flown directly at my head, just missing me. Just prior to that I had been wallowing in my discomfort over not having eaten for two days. The woodpecker's act instantly brought me out of my self-pitying stupor. Now I was present and ready to cleanse.

The sun had not struck the peak of Cadillac yet, but I could tell that it was going to be another nice day. As I sat facing Eagle Lake with my back to one of the trees, I closed my eyes and started my chakra cleansing. First I cleaned some nondescript sludge out of my base chakra, but when I reached into my sacrum, out came a baby. I marveled at what was happening. My love for this child was that of a mother—all-accepting. At the time I was sitting cross-legged, so I placed the child on my thigh and moved on to my solar plexus. After stopping my solar plexus chakra, I reached in and pulled out seven additional people who had had a great impact on my life. They included my father, my twin sister, my two daughters, my two wives, and a close friend. Then I realized that they were all stalkers. It was solely because of them that I had a firsthand knowledge of stalkerism.

By now the sun was rising over Cadillac. I could feel its warmth on my shoulders so I turned in greeting, thanked it for the new day, and brought its warmth and energy into my body before continuing. I needed to place something back into my solar plexus chakra to fill the void that had been created. I had taken out seven specific people who had tried to rule me with their wills, and now I needed to empower myself. Symbols were flashing in my mind. Solar = sun = spirit. Eagle = power of spirit. Eagle Lake . . . before me . . . stalker lessons . . . self- empowerment . . . solar plexus chakra. In my mind I created a triangle. First I ran a line from my solar plexus to the sun, then to Eagle Lake, then back to my solar plexus. Then I placed the essence of those symbols into my solar plexus and restarted my chakra.

I had been sitting in my sleeping bag for warmth, but now the day was getting hot. I imaginally picked up the child on my thigh, slipped out of my bag, and then replaced the child before continuing. As I cleansed my heart chakra another child came out, but this one was dead. It was accompanied by a spear, a sword, and a knife. I felt a great loss. I knew it was the me who had died emotionally at a very young age from the onslaught of my father (a great stalker teacher in my life). As I acknowledged the sorrow I was feeling, another part of me offered the child that had been birthed from my sacrum. I placed the new life back in my heart, and I marveled at the appropriateness of it all, to give birth anew and experience being reborn.

Just then two chickadees alighted nearby. I wondered if they were mates or just friends. I had always enjoyed their innocence, their curiosity, and their upbeat energy. Before continuing with my cleansing I made a vow to emulate them. When I got to my throat chakra I suddenly found myself standing next to "yokeman"—me in an alternate life in which I was enslaved. I had been tied to a yoke attached to a shaft that drew water from a deep well. The area was hot, dry, and dusty, and I spent my days walking in a circle, turning the shaft. I couldn't stand up straight, and my vertebrae were out of alignment, causing great pain. I was often whipped and given very little water, which made life unbearable. Seeing no way out of my dilemma, I was hopeless and despondent. Because this lifetime had never been resolved, I found that whenever I got into a controlling situation I would feel a great deal of pressure on the point of my spine where this yoke once sat. I realized that since I could feel my yokeman at those times, he must be able to feel me. I also knew that since our thoughts create our reality, the only way his situation was going to change was if he changed what he was sending out. Of course, he didn't know this, so I started sending him love, especially as he was making his presence known on my back. Now as I journeyed into his dimension, it appeared that his captors had abruptly vacated the scene. Only the "yokeman" was there, hanging from the yoke that he was tied to. Everything was quiet. I wondered if the invaders were still off chasing the former inhabitants. I found a hatchet and cut the ropes that bound my friend, carried him to a nearby dwelling, and placed him on a bed. He had dark curly hair, a dark beard, very blue eyes, and his only clothing was a loincloth. He was happy to see me and most appreciative of my help. A young woman appeared. I could tell she had been one of the servants. I couldn't see all of her face because she wore a cloth that covered her nose and mouth. Even so, she was very beautiful. I was quite drawn to her but I knew that she had come to help care for my friend, the yokeman, so I left him in her care.

I never did get my sixth and seventh chakras cleansed that day. Seeing the seven stalker teachers in my present life and resolving an enslavement issue in an alternate life had given me much to think about. Besides that, my third eye seemed to be functioning more than optimally at the time, so I decided to finish up later. It had come to me to take the time to individually thank each of the seven stalkers I had pulled out of my solar plexus for the lessons they had taught me. I was anxious to start this next phase.

Over the next two days I worked at bringing up each of the seven stalkers. I did a recapitulation of my life with each of them. I enumerated and thanked them for each lesson they had taught me concerning the world of the stalker, until I was able to beam each one with my heart. This cleansing was unlike most I had performed, in terms of its depth, vividness, and acuteness of personal symbolism. More often than not I was just pulling out sludgy material and various weapons that had been hurled at me by others or by myself. In retrospect, I don't think I could have accomplished this type of work had I not been receiving the energy of Eagle Lake spread before me.

A few weeks after my vision quest I decided to visit Eagle Lake at night. My intent was to attempt symbolically gazing with my left eye into the eagle's eye. The lake is shaped like an eagle (hence its name), and the remains of a hollow stump sit in the lake right where the eye in the eagle's head should be.

The stump still has some sprawling roots stretching out into the water towards the bank, and if you are agile, you can walk out on these to the stump. My intention was to position myself so that the moon, which symbolizes our subconscious, would be reflected in the water in the center of the stump. I was going to allow myself to journey into the moon's reflection, into the eye, to see what kind of information I could glean about the eagle and the third chakra.

First I became aware that standing on the lake was totally different from standing on the nearby land. While on the lake, I felt clear, focused, and self-empowered. I felt that I could focus my third eye to see into never-never land. As I looked back upon my previous visits to the lake, I could see that not only was the energy different on the water, but the two sides of the lake also had a different energy. In true hologrammatic form, as one entered the area from the tunnel by Eagle Lake Road and went to the right towards the eagle's head, the energy was very yang and masculine, while the energy on the left side of the lake was much softer and receptive, decidedly feminine. I noticed that I was more inclined to appreciate the surrounding woods on the left side, while the right put me more in my head. On the right side I was mainly interested in getting to my destination. I had lost interest in smelling the roses along the way.

CHAPTER 6

THE SACRAL CHAKRA: VALLEY COVE

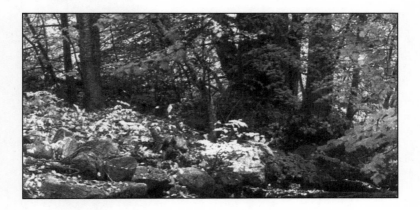

THE SACRAL CHAKRA is the region of emotions and feelings. Connected to our sexual organs, it pertains to both the quantity of sexual energy we may have and our ability to give and receive physical, mental, and spiritual pleasure. The chakra of our emotions and feelings, it is the connection to our lower self, or subconscious.

The sacral chakra on Mount Desert Island is located in Valley Cove on the southwest side of Somes Sound. An energetic doorway between the worlds here is conducive to journeying beyond the physical into other dimensions and lifetimes.

To reach Valley Cove take Route 102 south towards Southwest Harbor. As you enter Southwest Harbor, you will come down the long Carroll's Hill, past the small grocery mall on your left; then you will see Fernald Point Road on your left. Turn here and follow the road to the parking area for Valley Cove on your left. Just beyond the parking area is Valley Cove

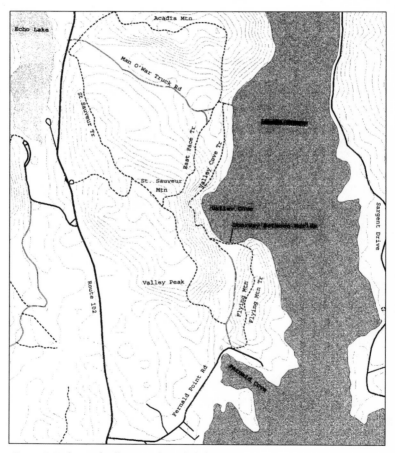

Figure 6: Trail Map of Valley Cove / Sacral Chakra

fire road. The beach at Valley Cove, which is your destination, is an easy half-mile walk down this road. A more scenic and entertaining route to Valley Cove is via Flying Mountain, which got its name from the Abnaki Indians. They believed the mountain originally flew off nearby St. Sauveur Mountain. Although short in length, the hike offers great views of both sides of Somes Sound and the Cranberry Islands just beyond the mouth of the Sound.

THE FLYING MOUNTAIN TRAIL (NPS rating: moderate; distance: .7 mile) leaves the east edge of the parking area where a cedar post marks the trailhead. From here it is about four hundred yards to the summit. The top has several large openings offering views across the Sound to Norumbega Mountain with Sargent Mountain behind it to the northeast, and the Cranberry Islands to the south. The grassy fields at the foot of the mountain were the site of the first Jesuit colony in 1613. The north side of the mountain offers a couple more spectacular overlooks before dropping steeply and quickly to the cove.

As you walk out onto the beach at the edge of the cove, you will be surrounded on your left by Valley Peak, the cliffs of St. Sauveur (which are probably the steepest on the island), and the two peaks of Acadia Mountain beyond that. The doorway itself is located to your left on the beach. Before seeking the doorway, become aware of how your body feels. Your low self is already aware of this doorway, so your body acts as an antennae. Keep observing your body as you walk. As you enter the doorway you will feel a change or a shift take place. I feel it as a pressure in the back of my neck and my head, but everybody senses energy differently. For example, some may feel it as heat, or pressure, or a tingling sensation somewhere in their body. Some may even have a visual effect. The secret is to notice a change, any change at all. You may not feel the doorway right away. Sometimes it takes a little time and practice to tune in. Try walking up and down the beach a few times while asking your low self for indications of the doorway's presence. If you are having trouble feeling the doorway, you will find it about one hundred feet west (to the left) of where you entered the beach from the Valley Cove fire road, at the mean high tide line.

The first time I encountered the doorway was on Halloween. I had decided to bike to Valley Cove and, needing a part, I stopped at a bike shop on my way. The owner asked where I was headed. I told him, "Valley Cove." His eyes widened. He leaned towards me and confided that he had heard that there was a doorway between the worlds there. This was auspicious, because Halloween is the day of the year when the veil between the worlds is the thinnest. Furthermore, when shop owners start talking about doorways between the worlds, you know a shift in consciousness and dimension is at hand. I headed out Fernald Point Road, then down the park road that leads to the cove. I dismounted my bike and, as I walked out onto the beach that surrounds half the cove, I allowed myself to slip into a feeling mode. I wanted to see if I could sense the raw change in the energy coming from the Earth indicating the presence of the doorway.

I began to notice a transition take place in my body as I neared a low group of rocks about halfway down the beach. I sat down on one of the rocks, closed my eyes, and listened. It felt good sitting in this energy field—soothing yet enlivening.

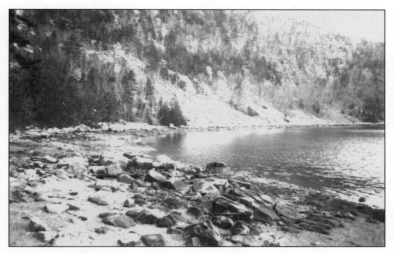

Valley Cove with Doorway Between the Worlds.

Since I wasn't getting any information, I opened my eyes and commenced dreamily to look at the beauty before me. Some sailors who had sought the peacefulness of the cove were anchored out before me. It was one of the last nice sailing days of the year. It was cosmic and idyllic, and as I breathed it in, I suddenly found myself looking down upon the whole scene. I saw a yin/yang symbol, the Chinese symbol for the duality. I realized that Somes Sound represents the sacral chakra. It had been sculpted out by glaciers—an incredible demonstration of yangness—yet it was filled with the Earth's most profound feminine symbol, the ocean. That was only the beginning. Just as the sacral chakra is linked to the reproductive system and represents the birth of the two sexes, the Earth on both sides of the Sound replicates the gender duality of our species. True to form, when looking at it as on a map, the feminine lies on the left side of Somes Sound, appropriately known as the "quiet side" of the island, and the masculine lies on the right.

First I saw the feminine side. The mouth to the Sound is a vaginal opening, Valley Cove the womb. This is especially appropriate because women also have a doorway between the worlds in their womb. The veil is the thinnest during their menses. It is a time of power when knowledge and information from the other side can be accessed. Just beyond Valley Cove is St. Sauveur, the belly of the woman, and Acadia Mountain, with its two peaks, the breasts. (Prior to intuiting this, I had always found Acadia Mountain a nurturing place to go.) To the north of this mountain lies Somesville, the head and the intellect. Somesville is a quiet New England village that stands on tradition. Just as in the development of the fetus, whereby the feminine precedes and supports the masculine, Somesville was the first village on Mount Desert Island.

On the other side of the Sound, looking north to south, I saw that Somes Sound symbolized a penis, with Somes Harbor and Somes Pond its two testicles. Norumbega Mountain is the body of the man, and Northeast Harbor manifests the head and intellect. Interestingly, Northeast Harbor is the most social of the exclusive wealthy enclaves on the island. After experiencing this phenomena, I began using the doorway in Valley Cove as a launching pad for shamanic journeys. I found I didn't have to be physically present in the doorway to benefit from its energy. Just picturing myself there is sufficient to facilitate a journey.

Two notable journeys that took place shortly after finding the doorway had to do with learning about the sun. A psychic had told me once that I had a sun in my aura, but she was unable to tell me why. She did say that the sun is the seat of fire, a transformational force that can be used to change what we don't like into what we want. This psychic also suggested that I journey to the sun, so that I could learn firsthand more about it.

A few days later I woke up in the middle of the night. My house is surrounded by woods and there wasn't a sound to be heard. I knew it was time to visit the sun, so I closed my eyes again and pictured myself back in the doorway in Valley Cove. I could see the beach and the rocks as clearly as if I were there. I stood looking into a hole between the rocks and asked for a guide to come out and help me.

Suddenly the bear appeared in front of me. I told him that I wanted to learn about the sun. He grabbed my hand, and the next thing I knew we were zooming through space, headed towards the sun. As I watched the sun, it kept getting larger and larger.

I kept thinking the bear was going to stop and point something out about the sun, but we just kept going right at it. As we shot into the flames of its corona, I remembered hearing once that the sun was pure love. I was musing over the timeliness of this information as we were engulfed in flames. It looked like hell, but it felt great, as if every cell of my body were being cleansed and titillated. Just as I decided to stay for a while, the experience started to fade. I thanked the bear for the trip and returned the way I had come.

It was another week before I journeyed again. Again I envisioned myself in Valley Cove. This time when I asked for a guide I got a cartoon coyote. I think I was being told to lighten up. I have a tendency to be too serious. It was a useful lesson, but I wasn't able to flow with old coyote that day. So I asked for the bear, and again he came. I had been told once that I and many others here now belonged to the Circle of the Sun. Wanting to know more about it, I asked the bear if he could teach me. This time he grabbed me by the hand and pulled me down into the earth. I had the sense of being sucked through a tunnel with earthen sides. Then suddenly I was standing in a stone tunnel with a barrier wall of stone just in front of me. I was aware of another presence on the other side of the wall, so I walked up to it and began peeling away layers. But instead of scaling rock, I suddenly was peeling a large onion. Then the onion became a book and I was turning its pages. I could now see the person on the other side of the stone wall. The barrier was still there, but I was able to see through it. The person looked as if he were made of crystals. He sparkled like sun when it glistens on the water. Suddenly I wasn't able to turn any more pages. I intuitively knew that more time needed to pass before I could come into contact with this crystalline man. Again, I thanked the bear and returned the way I had come.

A couple of weeks later, a friend told me that I should hike into Bald and Parkman Mountains. She promised magic. On the next fair day I went. I was carrying my daughter Christine on my back, and it wasn't long before she fell asleep to the rhythm of my walking. I, in turn, sank into the reverie of my mind. As I hiked along, the landscape blurred. Once again I saw the crystalline man behind the stone wall. When I had spied him on my shamanic journey, I just assumed he was an entity that I would learn more about at some future date. Now information was flooding towards me, telling me that the person I had seen behind the wall was actually me in the future, after I learned to embody my high self. I saw that the Circle of the Sun symbolized the act of continuously incarnating from your higher self (the sun) into the physical until you are able to embody that self in the physical domain. I was shown that many humans had done this in the past, and we were back here *en masse* to do it again as a gesture of the Second Coming. This was what the World of Unity was about. A feeling welled up from my gut to my heart and brought tears to my eyes. I was thankful to be alone as I hiked along crying softly to myself the tears of my joy and gratitude.

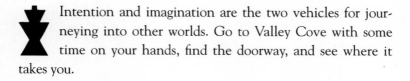 Intention and imagination are the two vehicles for journeying into other worlds. Go to Valley Cove with some time on your hands, find the doorway, and see where it takes you.

CHAPTER 7

THE BASE CHAKRA: WESTERN MOUNTAIN

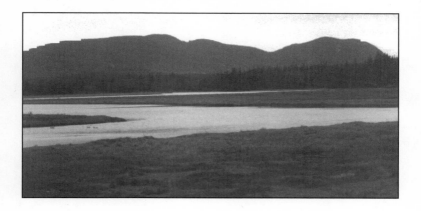

THE BASE CHAKRA is the one that grounds us to the physical. It is associated with physical sensation and physical functioning, also to survival and meeting our physical needs. The base chakra of Mount Desert Island is an unusual energy center in that it consists of two mountains, Mansell and Bernard, the first with a masculine tone, the latter feminine. They are referred to jointly as Western Mountain. Western Mountain is located between Long Pond and Seal Cove Pond on the "quiet side" of the island. Unlike the other mountains on Mount Desert whose peaks are rocky and

---

A view of the two peaks of Western Mountain, from Bass Harbor Marsh.

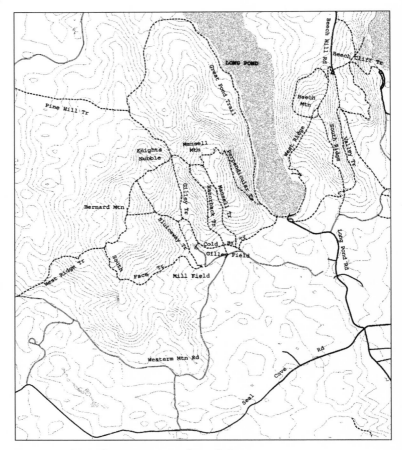

Figure 7: Trail Map of Western Mountain / Base Chakra

barren, those of Western Mountain are wooded. The energy here is primal and earthy. The woods in some places are so thick that they barely let light in. You will witness this primeval woodiness near the top of the South Face Trail, where the ground is a sea of moss.

Western Mountain has two main points of access, both of which can be reached from the Seal Cove Road. To reach the Seal Cove Road, take Route 102 south to Southwest Harbor. As you come into town you will see Seal Cove Road on your right. Turn right and go .5 mile up a hill to Long Pond Road on your right. Here you have two choices. You can go to the end of Long Pond Road, where there is a parking lot at the south end of Long Pond (sometimes referred to as Great Pond), or you can continue on Seal Cove Road to Western Mountain Road, where there is parking at both Gilley Field and Mill Field.

From the parking area at the south end of Long Pond, there is a number of trails that lead not only to Bernard and Mansell Mountains to the west of the pond, but also Beach Mountain (where you see the fire tower) to the east of Long Pond. The trailhead to Mansell and Bernard is marked by a cedar post located to the left behind the pumping station. All but the West Ridge Trail can be accessed from this point, although it is easier to reach the South Face and Sluiceway trails from Mill Field, and Mansell, Razorback and Gilley trails from Gilley Field. The West Ridge Trailhead is on the Western Mountain Road connector to Seal Pond, .2 mile on the right before the pond.

LONG POND TRAIL (NPS rating: easy; distance: 2.9 miles) provides two miles of easy walking along the edge of Long Pond before veering into the woods. Shortly you come to a small footbridge over Great Pond Brook. You may want to stop here for a few minutes and tune into the energy of the area. There is an energy vortex centered a little downstream of this bridge. Its periphery overlaps a portion of the bridge. Explore to see if you can find its center.

After the bridge, the trail becomes rougher as it ascends over exposed rocks and tree roots. At 2.9 miles the Long Pond Trail intersects the Western Trail, which continues another .4 mile to Great Notch at 949 feet. Here a signpost marks the intersection of several trails. Knights Nubble and Bernard Mountain are to the right where you can cut to the Sluiceway, South Face, and West Ridge trails; Gilley Field lies straight ahead via the Gilley Trail; and Mansell Mountain is to the left, from which you can divert to the Razorback, Mansell, and Perpendicular trails. All but the West Ridge Trail will take you back to the parking area at the pumping station. The Perpendicular Trail comes out on the Long Pond Trail about two hundred yards from the pumping station, while the others feed either directly or via Western Mountain Road (Sluiceway and South Ridge trails) onto the Cold Brook Trail, which also terminates on the Long Pond Trail just ten yards from the trailhead.

THE PERPENDICULAR TRAIL (NPS rating: strenuous; distance: 1.2 miles) and the Razorback Trail are both steep and strenuous climbs. The granite stairs up the first half of Perpendicular were built by the Civilian Conservation Corps, an amazing feat of craftsmanship. As they spiral up the east face of Mansell they offer spectacular views of Long Pond and Beach Mountain. The trail then enters the woods, skirts the base of a massive stone face, crosses a stream, and passes the trail's best overlook, a large stone slab that is a great spot for picnics. From here the trail continues to the top, which is so wooded there are no expansive views.

THE RAZORBACK TRAIL (NPS rating: strenuous; distance: .9 mile) follows the south ridge of Mansell. Its menu is the opposite of Perpendicular. Starting in the woods, it ascends steeply to rock slabs offering great views to the south. Western Mountain is known for its quiet wooded trails, and the Sluiceway and South Face trails epitomize this.

THE SLUICEWAY TRAIL (NPS rating: strenuous; distance: 1.1 miles), as its name implies, follows a stream for its entire length. It starts out gradually, then becomes consistently steep with often-tenuous footing on pine-needle-covered rocks and roots. After passing through Little Notch, for which the bakery in Southwest Harbor is named, it continues to the left to the peak of Bernard, where overlooks on either side of the trail provide outstanding vistas.

THE SOUTH FACE TRAIL (NPS rating: strenuous; distance: 1.7 miles) also climbs steadily through a variety of woods as it rounds the west side of the mountain. About halfway up, the West Ridge Trail branches off to the left. As you continue to the right, the South Face Trail becomes more gradual, finally entering a thickly wooded area whose hillsides are covered with moss, giving the appearance of a place where fairies and gnomes abound. Perhaps you can find a doorway here.

THE WEST RIDGE TRAIL (NPS rating: strenuous; distance: 1.1 miles) runs off Western Mountain Road about .2 mile before it reaches Seal Cove Pond. The trailhead is marked on the right of the road by a cedar post, and there is a small dirt pull-off on the left that will accommodate two to three cars. This trail has some steep rocky sections interspersed with moderate wooded sections. Shortly before joining the South Face Trail, it opens into some large rocky fields with scattered clumps of trees and occasional standing stones perched as sentinels guarding end-less views to the south and west.

Although these trails are all fun and quite spectacular to hike, I find getting off the trails and exploring the woods more satisfying, though the Park Service discourages this on account of unexpected drops. Walk consciously. My first off-trail venture into the base chakra was on Mansell one morning several years ago. No sooner had I started up the Perpendicular Trail than I heard an inner voice telling me, "Leave the trail!" It complained that the trail was sterile, that I wouldn't find true adventure there. I love hiking this trail, so I was hesitant to leave it, but after several false starts I relented and headed up the steep slope into the woods. I always assume I am called into the woods for a reason, so I continued to let my intuition lead me as I climbed higher and deeper into the woods. As I approached what I felt was the midpoint on the mountain, the terrain became moderate and rolling with large outcroppings of rock here and there. The woods at this point were less dense, with a mixture of deciduous and evergreen trees. As I came around a large hummock, I was attracted to a rock about six feet in height that had the distinct profile of a human head. Intrigued by this, I climbed onto the rock to tune in and greet it.

At first the rock told me that it had been waiting for me, and it was happy to see me. I was a little confused by this because I had never noticed this rock before. How could the rock have been waiting for me, let alone know that I was even alive? I gave up any rational approach, closed my eyes again,

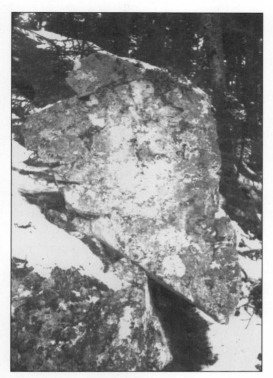

Talking Rock on Mansell Mountain.

and just listened. Next I heard the rock murmuring, "We are all one." The words floated through my head, accompanied by a light and a warm radiance that suffused my heart. Then the rock told me that I didn't need to come physically to it in order to make contact or talk. It would be with me the moment I closed my eyes and pictured it. To this day this "Head Rock" remains a source of grounding for me. I recommend finding a rock spirit to connect to your base chakra.

That fall I decided to do a four-day vision quest on Mansell. It was a dreary day, end of September, hovering between rain and snow. Only six weeks had passed since my last vision quest, but I was feeling the call to be on the land again. This was my seventh quest on Mount Desert Island in five years, and for the first time I was questing on the base chakra of the island. My intent was to ground my light body into the physical domain.

It started to rain lightly as I climbed up the Perpendicular Trail. I had toyed with the notion of questing on Bernard Mountain, Mansell's feminine counterpart, but spirit kept nudging me towards Mansell. I should have known this was going to be a difficult passage. By the time I found a suitable site it was pouring. Normally I would have chosen an inconspicuous spot, but the woods seemed so dark and dreary that I decided to encamp at the edge of a clearing overlooking Long Pond. I was soaked by the time I got my shelter erected. With only a tent, a sleeping bag, water, and the clothes on my back, I stripped, climbed into my bag, and snuggled there for four days.

I was looking forward to four days of peace and light, but almost immediately I started to get a right-sided migraine. Originating at the base of my skull, it encompassed the right side of my head, then centered in my right eye. Concurrent with the headache, I had the sensation of three people in my body, all striving for attention. Two men, Jeff and Allen, symbolized the two poles of my male side—Jeff as arrogance, and Allen as indecision. Paul, a friend with AIDS, represented both poles of my female side, creativity and fear. Of the three, I was closest to Paul.

Right-sided headaches were not new for me. I had been having them once or twice a month for a year; they usually lasted three days. To me they represented left-brain dominance symbolically danced out in my head, a throwback to my overbearing patriarchal upbringing. During one of my previous head/eye-aches I had noticed that several points in my eye hurt. As I went into one of the points, I saw first a door in front of me a little to my left. The door was holding back a throbbing and pushing mass of humanity. As I looked at the door I felt extreme fear. It was slightly ajar, and there were fingers wrapped around its entire edge. The door was pulsating even as the clamoring masses strained to open it wider. I knew it was only a matter of time before they got in. I also knew that when that time came, I would be obliterated. There was nowhere to go. As panic hit me, I became Paul. I realized that I was experiencing the suffocating fear of AIDS. Several other points of pain spangled in my right eye, each attached to a particular onslaught from the World of Separation. The pain was so great I couldn't go fully into each one. As I lay writhing in my sleeping bag, I tried everything I knew to drive these energies out of my body, and the pain out of my head. Nothing seemed to work. I kept calling inwardly for help. All I heard was, "Use your imagination." This just made me angry. I was feeling too much pain to feel creative.

On the morning of the fourth day I decided to try a creative approach I'd recently learned. Boogie-busting is a technique for helping disembodied entities locate the light. We may well have various entities in us who, for one reason or another, have contracted with us to be there. These beings never went into the light when they died; now they want a body to enjoy the pleasures of life and work out their unfinished business. We, for our part, have certain difficulties that their personalities or strengths compensate for. For instance, if my will had been broken, I might attract a very assertive entity. In boogie-busting there really is no such thing as the battle between good and evil, angel and devil. We are all earnest beings journeying towards the light. We the living just need to help these non-embodied entities along. The exercise involves imagining a tunnel with a bright light at the other end. You become aware of who is next to you (internally). As each entity makes itself known, you acknowledge them, thank them for their help and the lessons shared, and state that you no longer need them. Then you ask them if there is anything you can do to honor them and help them on their way. After carrying out their request, you escort them down the tunnel and into the light.

As I created my tunnel and attuned to who was in my space, I got the impression that I was the door-keeper for the whole throbbing mass of humanity that had its fingers wrapped around the edge of the door in my earlier vision. They were collectively screaming to go to the light. Because I was the door-keeper, they felt they had to go through my body. I started to aid some of them but, as I looked at the endless line to my right waiting to get through me, I became outraged at their imposition on me. I was hungry and tired, and my head hurt. I didn't have the patience for this. I kept thinking, why do these people have to go through me? Why can't they find the light themselves? All they have to do is look up! At the point my anger climaxed I reached up and grabbed the veil of the universe above me, ripped it open, and yelled, "CAN'T YOU SEE IT? IT'S RIGHT THERE!" Suddenly a flood of brilliance hit my face and warmed my body. It felt so . . . good. Then I realized that my headache was gone.

Another year went by before I was drawn to quest on Western Mountain again. I had recently attempted to manifest a vision quest to California, and it had not come to pass. First, I had created an elaborate picture of my trip and imbued it with a lot of fun energy. I even had my bags packed, but something, some inner character, was blocking the fulfillment of my calling. I could have this grail; all I had to do was to open my heart. I therefore decided to go out on the south face of

Bernard Mountain, the feminine aspect of the base chakra, to see if I could not only open my heart there, but ground physical abundance and prosperity as well.

The timing for this quest was ideal. It was fall; the full moon was near. It was a time of harvest and fulfillment. In all my previous quests I had gone the duration without eating, but I had recently been reading Thich Nhat Hanh's account of the life of Buddha, where the Vietnamese monk points out that you don't need to cannibalize your body in order to achieve enlightenment. So I decided that, rather than fast for four days, I would allow myself a slice of bread with molasses on it three times a day. This proved quite beneficial. It dispelled a lot of the discomfort and imbalance of starvation and allowed me to attend to my inner journey more fully.

After finding a suitable site I discreetly set up my tent in the shelter of some trees. Then I designated a circle that would be the boundary of my existence for the next four days. I included in my circle not only my tent, but a nearby rock that was shaped like an old wooden coffin—just large enough to lie out on, with a view of the ocean to the south and west. I briefly pondered the significance of the rock's shape, then put it out of my mind. It was an ideal location for sunsets; it also corresponded to the west on the medicine wheel, the direction of introspection. My circle was at the edge of a large field, about five acres in size, that was strewn with boulders with an occasional clump of trees. There were also standing stones here and there, some four to five feet tall, like sentinels guarding the field. They appeared lost in thought as they gazed out to the oceanic horizon. As I sat in awe of the landscape about me, I took out a bag of corn meal that I had brought with me and gave thanks to the six directions by scattering the corn. I stated my intentions for being there, and asked for help and guidance on my journey to meet myself.

My first day I sat outside soaking in the sun, doing occasional yoga and Chi Kung exercises to relax and improve the flow of my energy. I sat for long periods with my eyes closed, observing my breath and my thoughts and feelings. My experience with Alchemical Hypnotherapy has taught me that our low self, or subconscious, is made up of a cast of characters. By getting to know these characters, you get to know yourself. You can also work with them to create change in your life. These are not ghosts or spirits. They are selves, characters of us in our life drama.

As I watched my inner dance, I noticed two familiar women who kept popping up. They seemed anguished and in need of my attention. One was quite persistent. At first I thought my low self was attracted to this person because she is quite pretty, so I kept dismissing her. But as she persisted in coming up, I finally asked why. I hardly knew this person, having met her for the first time just three months earlier. Still my low self seemed intent on wanting to show me something about her, so I gave him free rein and watched. As I reran the tape of that afternoon when the female character first appeared, I suddenly remembered a look that this woman had given me. It had been very brief, but she had suddenly dropped all pretenses and given me a searching look that I felt in my soul. As I felt her gaze once again tugging at me, I realized that she was doing something that I often did, especially with women. Having lost touch with our high selves, she and I had the same habit of searching outside ourselves for a heartful connection to represent the divine. And although such a link can be found, I knew it was as ephemeral and fleeting as the look she gave me compared to the profundity that lies within. Becoming conscious of this character helped me to redirect myself inward.

As I continued to work down through the layers of my armoring and to open my heart, I kept banging up against a despondent, depressed feeling. It was a sorrow that I was very accustomed to, so much so that I had learned to ignore it to the point of not feeling it. But now that the door to this character was open, I realized I was imbued with it. It was time to venture in and meet who was there.

It had rained considerably the second day, been overcast and drizzly the third, and now on the morning of the fourth day, it was wet and cloudy. My extended stay in my tent had driven me far inward. I felt a strong connection to my heart and my inner guides, and I was readily getting answers to questions concerning feelings that were mushrooming up in my body.

I was being taken back to the first four years of my life, a time that I had blocked from my memory. A few years ago a friend reading my astrological chart had told me that I had come into the world on a very tyrannical energy, analogous to being held face down in the mud, without being able to move.

I heard a sound outside. Curious, I quietly pulled back the flap of my tent. Standing twenty feet away, oblivious to my presence, was a doe nibbling on some bushes. She looked healthy and strong. Occasionally she would nervously raise her head, her ears quivering, looking for danger. I watched her for several minutes until something beyond my awareness sent her fleeing into the nearby woods. I recalled that the deer symbolized gentleness. I felt certain she had come to remind me to be gentle with myself as I ventured inward. As I sank back into the feelings that were welling up, I found myself in a room that was pervasively oppressive. I felt afraid and vulnerable. I had the impression that the ceiling in the room was a black ominous cloud that kept bearing down on me. It was a relentless pressure that I had to constantly battle against. It was hard for me even to hold my head up. I wanted to stand up straight but I kept sagging from the weight, especially my left side. I could see two characters emerging from myself. They were "Nobody Likes Me" and "I'm Not Worthy." They had influenced and colored much of my life.

I reached in and gathered my young selves to me. As I held them to my bosom, I promised them that I would protect and watch over them. I sent them love. They told me their story of how they had tried to be good and worthwhile, yet no matter how much they did, or how hard they tried, it was never enough. Nobody liked them and they felt doomed to failure. Again that same despondent, depressed feeling returned. I told them that prosperity was not a result of how hard you worked but a state of consciousness. What we really needed to do was to stop sending out our doomed feelings, to relax and open our hearts.

By evening most of the clouds had cleared. I went out and sat on my rock and watched as the sun turned the remaining clouds red, pink, orange, and purple. I was feeling vital and alive. I was excited about the work I had done with my inner characters; my confidence was soaring. Just as the sun was settling on the horizon, I looked it square in the eye and affirmed prosperity into my life.

That night I crawled longingly into my sleeping bag. I was looking forward to spending more time with my inner characters. But as I tuned in I got overwhelmed with a multitude of pain that bounced from one part of my body to another. I tried everything I knew to release these feelings but nothing worked. Finally, after four or five hours, I gave up. I couldn't sleep, so I climbed out of my tent and took a deep breath of the cool, fall air. The clouds had cleared and the stars sparkled brilliantly in the sky. The moon was just setting to the west over Blue Hill Bay, creating a path of light on the water. As I relaxed and melted into the beauty of the night, it suddenly occurred to me what I was doing wrong. I had been trying to stop and evict the feelings that belonged to my two most recent characters. To them it was just more of the same treatment they had always received. I remembered a song that is sung at the closing of the Maine Healing Arts Festival each year. It is a Sufi song. Everyone at the festival forms two circles, one inside the other, facing each other. We then sing individually to each person in the opposing circle:

"Listen listen listen to my heart song,
Listen listen listen to my heart song,
   I will never forget you,
   I will never forsake you,
   I will never forget you,
   I will never forsake you."

I added my own closing line, "I accept you."

It had been another four days of hard internal work, facing hunger and periods of intense monotony, as I sorted through a myriad of overwhelming feelings searching for the underlying characters. But it had been more than worth it. These characters had been a drain on my energy for a long time. With the facilitating aid of the base chakra, I had broken through and unified the most debilitating parts of myself.

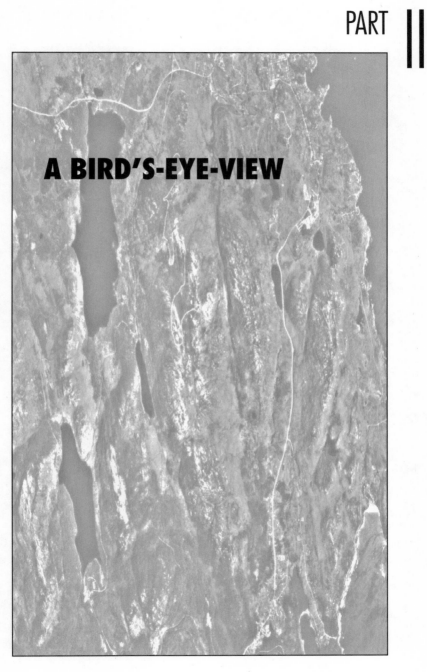

PART II

A BIRD'S-EYE-VIEW

SATELLITE VIEWS OF MOUNT DESERT ISLAND

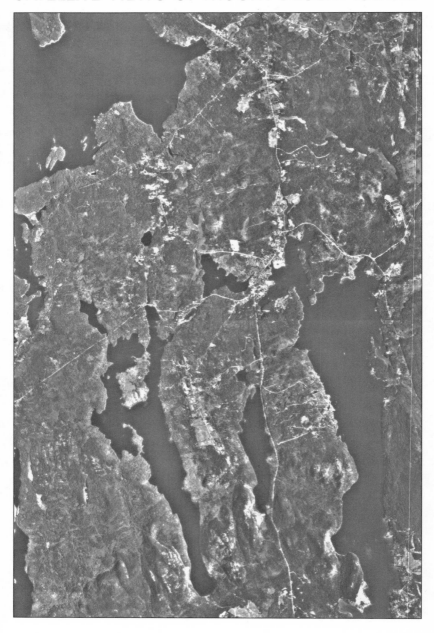

Long Pond (on left), Echo Lake and Somes Sound. The Base Chakra (Western Mountain) is to the left of Long Pond.

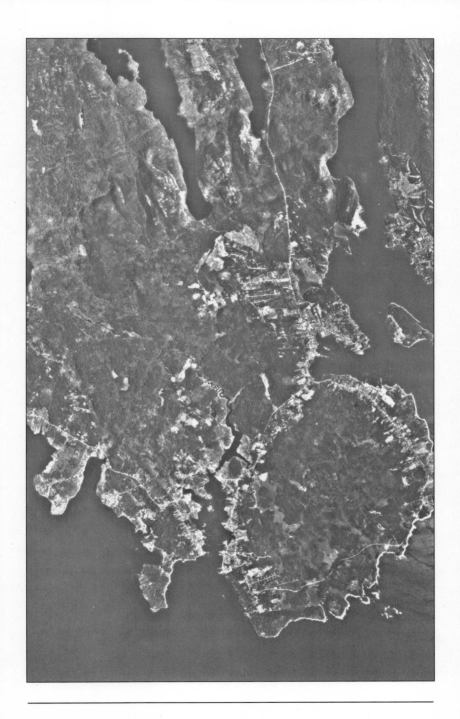

Southwest Harbor, Bass Harbor and Seawall.

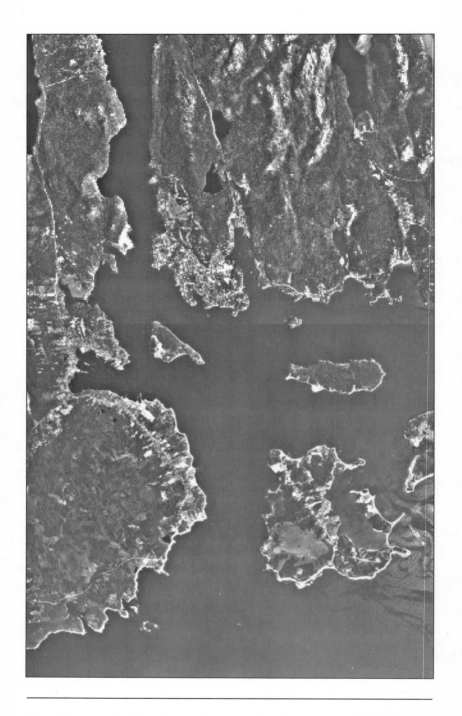

98 *The mouth of Southwest Harbor and Somes Sound, with Greening, Sutton and Cranberry Islands.*

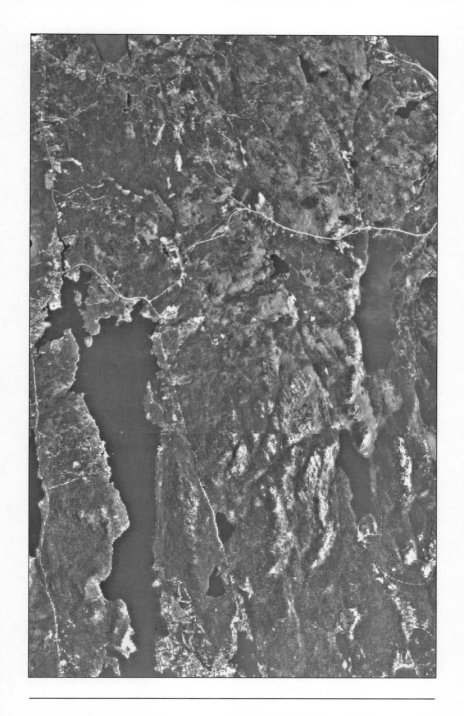

Sargent Mountain, with Somes Sound (Sacral Chakra) to the left and Eagle Lake (Solar Plexus Chakra) to the right.

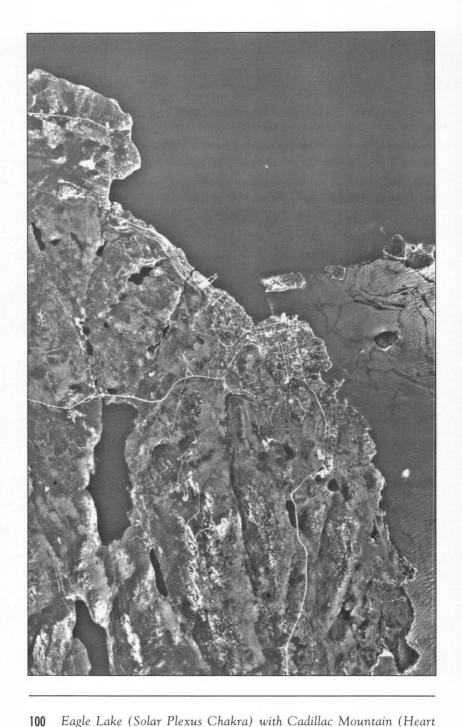

100   *Eagle Lake (Solar Plexus Chakra) with Cadillac Mountain (Heart Chakra) to the east and Bar Harbor to the northeast.*

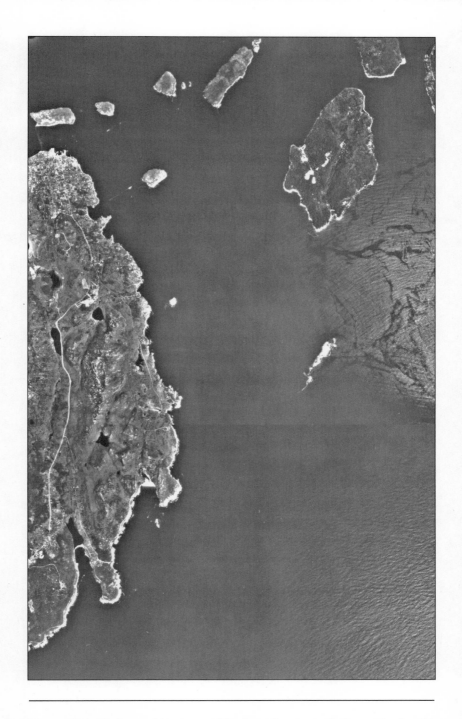

View of Bar Harbor and Porcupine Islands at the top, with Great Head 101
and Sand Beach (Throat, Brow, and Crown Chakras) below.

PART III

THE
SEVEN CHAKRAS
ON CADILLAC MOUNTAIN

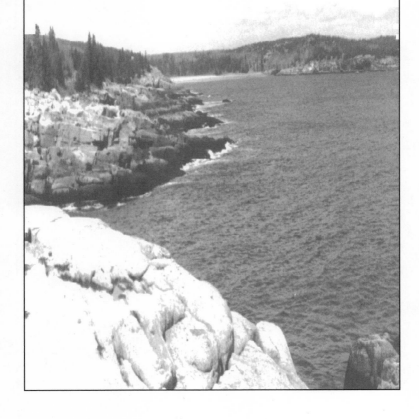

CHAPTER 8

THE BASE CHAKRA
OF CADILLAC MOUNTAIN:
THE "WOLFIE" ROCK

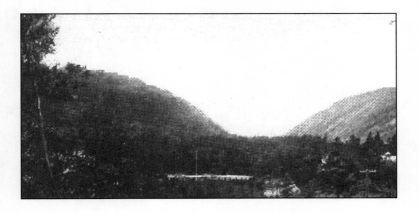

THE BASE CHAKRA on the south ridge of Cadillac Mountain is a large rock located along the section of the South Ridge Trail that runs between Blackwoods Campground and Route 3. From the trailhead in Blackwoods Campground, go about .1 mile to where you see a number of worn pathways wandering off to the left of the trail. The rock, the size of four cars stacked two on two, is located about forty yards to the left of the trail. There is a circle of stones in the ground on the far side of the rock. If you stand in the circle and face the rock, you will notice a face.

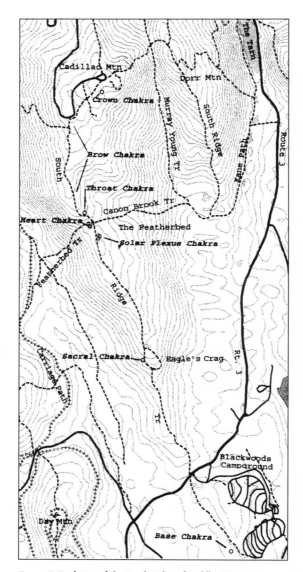

Figure 8: Trail Map of the South Ridge of Cadillac Mountain
        Base Chakra

Another approach to the rock comes from Route 3. It is a pleasant half-mile walk through the woods. The trailhead is located one hundred yards south of the entrance to Blackwoods Campground on the same side of the road. Since there are no real markers to the rock, I suggest that you key your low self to tell you when you get to it. Otherwise, keep looking down to the right when you feel you are getting near. You will find that you can see the rock better through the woods after you have gone slightly beyond it. It is the only rock of its size that is visible from the trail. If you suddenly find yourself at the campground, retrace your steps.

My first encounter with the rock happened one day several years ago when I ran into some friends, Ed and Patti, in Bar Harbor. They had just heard from a woman friend about a rock at the base of Cadillac that had an eye on it, and they were anxious to share the news. They told me there was also a circle of stones, possibly a medicine wheel, near the rock. According to their friend the rock had spoken prophetically to her. Ed urged me to go check it out. Ed's directions to the rock were from Blackwoods Campground, but since I was coming from the opposite direction, I asked my low self to alert me to its presence. Sure enough, even though the rock was in the woods, forty yards off the trail, I knew the instant I came upon it.

As I walked around the rock I noticed the circle of stones about twenty feet away. The stones were covered with moss, and you could tell that they had been there a long time. I first checked to see if the circle was a medicine wheel, but the rocks didn't line up with the four directions and I couldn't discern any energy field above the circle, which medicine wheels create. But as I looked at the rock from the circle I noticed a very distinct face in it. It was startling. In fact, the rock was a

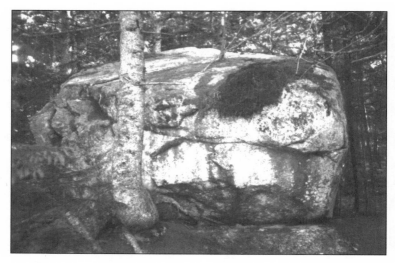

"Wolfie Rock"—Base Chakra on the south ridge of Cadillac, located next to Blackwoods Campground.

great big head. So I decided that the circle was a point of observation. As I viewed the face, I saw that there were Christmas ferns growing on the top of the rock that represented the hair. The chin was receding, which gave the countenance a childlike demeanor, completely free of arrogance. The right eye, representing the island of reason, was ferociously discerning, while the left eye, which was much larger and represented the island of silent knowledge, seemed to contain the universe. Only in the left eye were there different sizes and colors of lichen and moss. From the circle it was like looking at a Rorschach test. As I stared into the large eye I saw an endless parade of images and faces. With its wise yet innocent demeanor, the rock also reminded me of my son, so I started referring to it as the Wolfie (his nickname) Rock.

After staring at the face and left eye for a while, I decided to climb up onto the rock to what would be the crown chakra of the head. After getting comfortable, I tuned in to the energy of the rock, which was flowing through me. I then asked the rock if it wished to tell me anything, and I began to observe the mental impressions that flowed through me.

The first impression I received was that the rock could heal Mary. A twenty-seven-year-old nurse with a six-year-old son, Mary was the daughter of Wendell, a friend of mine. After she had started having seizures two weeks before, it was discovered that she had a tumor in the right side of her brain. Having been schooled with the "attack the foreign substance" approach of Western medicine, Mary announced even before a treatment modality had been arrived at that she wanted to take an aggressive approach. To those trained in discerning the balance between the inner male and female, it was fairly evident that Mary's inner male was calling the shots and had a death grip on her inner female. The rock showed me that Mary needed to slow down. She was in "super beta" and she needed to be in theta, which would put her one-on-one with her feminine side. Since this rock was a power spot, it was like a super-resonator for the theta brainwave, which would help Mary if she would spend time there.

Wendell crossed my path the next day and updated me about Mary, and I, in turn, told him about the rock. The following Tuesday, Wendell, Mary, Wendell's ex-wife Sue, and I went to the rock. Since what we were doing was new to Mary and Sue, I kept it simple and just told them about the importance of resonating at theta. I also gave her my chapter, "I Am the Mountain," hoping it would help her relate to the rock and nature, and guide her thinking towards self-empowerment.

I wanted to give her some time with this before introducing the inner male and female, the need for balance between the two, and how the consequence of her imbalance was reflected in herself and the people around her.

The summer progressed. Mary had the tumor removed from her head. She also became buddies with the rock to the extent that, on the night before her checkup to see how she was progressing postoperatively, the rock came to her in her dreams. She told me that she found herself approaching the face when suddenly she stopped. Her husband behind her urged her to continue, but she told him she had to wait. Suddenly a bear appeared. Her husband gasped and grabbed her to run away, but she held her ground and said, "Chris has taught me not to fear the bear." (She evidently had read my chapter on the mountain.) The bear then came to her, picked her up, carried her to the rock, and placed her on it, at which point she felt a soothing energy run through her body. Then she awoke knowing everything was going to be all right.

This is just one of a growing number of stories surrounding the Wolfie Rock. Each one is singular, each unique. During Mary's ordeal, Wendell's wife Annie made her own pilgrimage to the rock because she had a great deal of disruptive rage about some things. She was leaning against the rock with her hands and when she pulled away, not one, but two flakes broke away in the shapes of hearts (the scars of which can still be seen), telling her she needed to view the world through her fourth, not her third, chakra. Annie, in turn, told a woman who came into her stained-glass studio in Southwest Harbor about the rock. The woman wrote back saying, "After I left your store, the very next day I found 'Wolfie.' As I speak I can feel his heartbeat. It was one of the most powerful earthspots I have been to. I could hear the sound and rhythm radiating out of 'Wolfie.'. . . I close my eyes anywhere I am now and can be right there again. Thank you!"

Meanwhile, I was learning from the rock that it represented the doorway to the base chakra on the south ridge. The base chakra is our connection to the physical, the Earth, and I saw that the rock is the head of a child because that is how we first manifest in the physical. And like this rock, a child is all-knowing. They are born in a delta brainwave. They are sheer spirit.

CHAPTER 9

THE SACRAL CHAKRA OF CADILLAC MOUNTAIN: THE CRACK IN THE COSMIC EGG

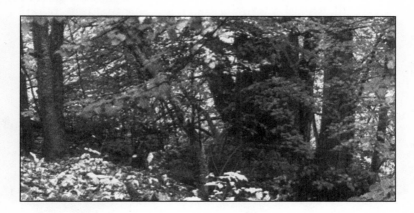

WHILE I WAS SPENDING a lot of time walking on the south ridge of Cadillac, the mountain also showed me several of its other chakra centers. The entrance to the second chakra is signaled by three stones located just to the left of the trail about halfway between the two intersections with the Eagle's Crag Loop (approximately one mile from Route 3). The center of the three is seven feet tall and looks like an egg that has been split open, an interesting embodiment for the chakra of sexual relationships. The other two rocks symbolize the two extremes of behavior found in the

World of Separation. One rock is the head of a bulldog representing arrogance, and the other rock (on the upper left corner) is a rabbit in full flight representing fear.

On one of my journeys to the island of silent knowledge I was shown how the epitome of these two extremes is being played out in the physical. It was the beginning of January, and I had just finished building a wood-fired sauna. Saunas are conducive to journeying, so I was anxious to try mine out. I had recently met Paul (see Chapter 7) and learned that he had AIDS and, while I was in my sauna, he came to my attention. As I scanned him with my inner vision and attempted to connect with him energetically, I realized that he had many walls. No matter what approach I took to communicate with him, he would block it. I sensed that he was fed up with all those

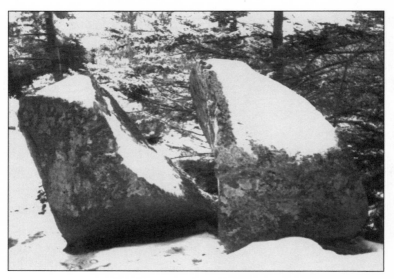

"Crack in the Cosmic Egg," Sacral Chakra on the South Ridge of Cadillac Mountain.

approaches. In fact, he seemed disgusted. Finally I gave up trying to transmit any type of consolation, help, or even healing
intent, and just tried connecting our hearts. When I pictured
him, I said the words, "From my heart to your heart may love
abide." I felt him completely relax and open to my presence.
Then I saw that Paul was disgusted with the way the will
(male) had been projected without the heart during the World
of Separation, and he was therefore retaliating by opting not
to use his will. In a symbolic bodily gesture, he had so completely surrendered his will to the point that he was refusing to
lift even one single antibody in his defense.

In terms of the balance between the will and the heart,
AIDS (fear) is the counterbalancing result of having gone to
the extreme of dropping the atomic bombs (arrogance).
Dropping the bomb was the epitome of the will without the
heart, and now we have the epitome of the heart without
the will.

Don Alberto, a Shuar native of Ecuador, claims that the
imbalance created in the world can be turned around in a gen-
eration. All we have to do is seed a new dream. As Don
Alberto told John Perkins in his book *The World Is As You
Dream It,* "Your people dreamed of huge factories, tall build-
ings, as many cars as there are raindrops in this river. Now you
begin to see that your dream is a nightmare." Don Alberto
bent to pick up a stone. "The problem is your country is like
this stone." He threw it far into the river. "Everything you do
ripples across the Mother."

I think that in order to seed a new dream, we need to dis-
cover the path we came here to walk.

In December of 1988 I reached a point in my life where nothing was working out. I had spent years creating a picture of what I thought I wanted, but once I had it, it felt empty. So one day I went out into my yard, sat on a large rock, and expressed my emptiness to God. I told him that I felt I was here for a reason, and I was ready to walk the path that I had come to walk. One week later my life began to change. At first there was a dramatic upheaval which left no doubts in my mind that I was on a new path. I entered the transition. Over a period of two years I went from being a pharmaceutical salesman to an explorer and journeyer among chakras. This didn't happen all at once. It was a process of undoing the old world and opening to a new one. The process continues. I guarantee you that if you ask from your heart to walk your path, two things are going to happen: you're going to get danced through your false programs, and you're going to find out who you are.

THE SOLAR PLEXUS CHAKRA OF CADILLAC MOUNTAIN: THE BALANCE POINT

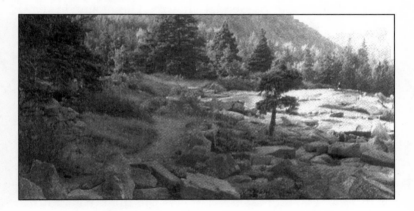

THE THIRD CHAKRA on the south ridge of Cadillac is located at the knoll that lies just to the south of the Featherbed, overlooking it (2.4 miles from Route 3). As mentioned, not only is the pond that lies in the Featherbed (where I was embraced by the bear) in the shape of a heart, but there are two adjoining knolls, one on either side of it, that represent breasts. True to form, the left breast is round and full, very feminine, while the right one is smaller and knobbier, more masculine-looking. Intuiting this though, created a problem, because I had been separately shown that the right breast was also the third chakra on the mountain, and I couldn't figure out why that one knoll represented both a male and a female aspect.

Then Wendell stopped in one day. He had returned two days prior from Mary's operation (see Chapter 8) and, having heard me talk about the south ridge of Cadillac, decided to climb it. His intent was to go to the top, but he got only as far as a knoll that overlooked a grassy field. He tried to go further but was called back to the knoll by his inner voice. He was informed that he had gone far enough. The mountain urged him to be present, to absorb the essence of the place and the moment.

I knew the grassy field Wendell was talking about. In the summer a hollow-core grass grows up out of the pond to a height of about three feet. Many times, especially during my last quest, I had sat and watched the wind as it swirled and danced with the grass. I had also been amused by the expression of green, since it is the color of the heart chakra.

Wendell had spent the last five years saving his three children from various disasters. Mary was the third. He said that he felt as if he had taken the three of them out in a canoe without life jackets. The canoe had capsized, none of them could swim, and it had been a life-and-death struggle to save them and get them to shore.

Suddenly I realized that Wendell was bringing me a gift of insight, and I told him that, by having him stop on that knoll, the mountain was congratulating him. Then I raised my right arm so my fist was a foot in front of my face and told him that he had walked to the power center of the mountain, which symbolized his male side. I laid my left hand over my right fist and told him that it was also the right breast, symbolizing his feminine side. By drawing Wendell to that point—the one place where the masculine and the feminine fuse—the mountain was telling him that through his efforts to save his children he had achieved a balance between his inner male and female. I thereby dubbed the knoll "The Balance Point," finally understanding how it manifested as Cadillac's solar plexus chakra.

CHAPTER 11

THE HEART CHAKRA OF CADILLAC MOUNTAIN: THE POND

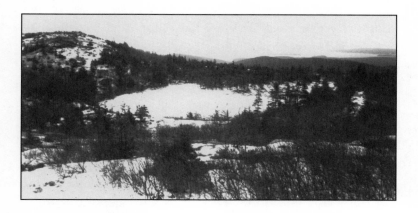

THE FOURTH CHAKRA on the mountain is the heart-shaped pond about 2.5 miles up the south ridge, and a little over a mile below the summit. This was where I experienced being embraced by the bear.

My first apperception that the pond was the heart chakra on the mountain happened almost a year to the day after being embraced by the bear. I had recently come back from Hawaii, where I spent time exploring Haleakala, the heart chakra for the Hawaiian Islands. I decided to hike the south ridge of Cadillac. When I reached the Featherbed, I walked out onto

---

The Heart Chakra on Cadillac Mountain—the Heart Shaped Pond.

the pond and was charting its circumference when I suddenly heard the words "heart chakra" whispered in my ear. As I looked around, I noticed the heart shape in the pond. Then I saw the two knolls on either side, like two breasts, and that really got me laughing.

To sit on the mountain, especially at its heart center, greatly enhances one's ability to feel, just as it did the day I stood on the pond and did my sun meditation. I have journeyed many times, sat for the day at the edge of the pond, and come away centered in my heart and my knowingness. I call it a day of processing. I get in touch with my low self and let it express its feelings and its confusion about people I've encountered, discussions I've had, and telepathic impressions I've picked up and wasn't cognizant of. I gently untie the knots of confusion until I am able to glow. Spending several days at the heart center extends my ability to feel literally millions of miles into the physical dimension, and beyond that into other dimensions. The physical world becomes the world of energy. Each morning I know exactly when the sun is cresting the horizon because I can feel it as a glow in my heart. It is a wonderful way to be greeted. I also feel the moon rising each night in my body. The lunar body, being connected to my subconscious, allows me to see where I am blocking the flow of energy in my body, where my belief system collides with my feelings and becomes congested knots. I then do the work to untie them.

During a vision quest one February I fasted at the edge of the pond for seven days and spent time working on my right knee. It was so cramped with repressed feelings that I had stopped running a year before because of the pain. I viewed this as my inability to walk in my maleness. While I was at the nucleus of the heart chakra, I was able to feel energy with a clarity that I had never experienced before.

As I worked on my knees I was astounded at how much I was able to move out of them without overloading the rest of my body. As each release occurred, I followed exactly where the energy was going and, if it started to get bogged down in any part of my body, I invariably found I could relax that part and mentally direct the energy along. I also found that I could extend my energy fingers and rake them through my body, moving energy along that way too. The whole time, I was being directed. Each time I placed one of the pointed dowels that I was using to release the blocks, I would be shown via a tickling sensation where the next placement was to be. Appreciating the advantage I was being given, I spent several hours each day moving massive amounts of blocked energy. I also began to experience other lifetimes impacting on my knee. They were lifetimes of control in the World of Separation where I had been persecuted for living my truth. They were lifetimes that had been left unresolved and thus set the stage for my present situation (see Chapter 5). Now I was being given not only the chance to resolve them, but a way to do it in a breathtakingly accelerated fashion.

As the end of my week drew near and I cleared channels in my body, I found that I was able to light up my heart as I had never done before. My ability to connect energetically with others made it seem as if they were right next to me, even if they were thousands of miles away. Information also became readily available. True to its name, the island of silent knowledge was plugging into the psychic, interdimensional, worldwide web.

On the last day of my quest, I began to see a trinity of heart symbols. I found I was sitting next to a pond in the shape of a heart, on a mountain that activated people's hearts; the mountain, in turn, besides being touched first in the United States by the sun, is on an island that is in the shape of a human heart. As I pondered the magnitude of this progression, I became curious as to how much of the Earth would be influenced by this mountain as it was activated. Upon asking, I was shown two pointer fingers side by side. Then they separated, and each drew a semi-circle in front of me, one facing the other. They joined again at the bottom, completing a circle. It was the whole Earth.

CHAPTER 12

THE THROAT, BROW, AND CROWN CHAKRAS OF CADILLAC MOUNTAIN: THE VIEW FROM HERE

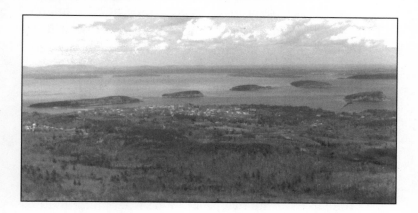

IF WE SWITCH OUR VISION from seeing to looking and view the upper part of the south ridge in a linear fashion, it becomes evident that the knoll, or left breast, that is to the north of the pond is a chin, making the side of the knoll the throat chakra. This is the first of the top three chakras, all of which are feminine. Although the throat is the most masculine of the three, having to do with outward expression, it lies on a very feminine aspect on the mountain.

View from the top of Cadillac Mountain.

The view from this knoll, surrounded by mountains, ocean, and islands, is exhilarating. To see and feel the heart and third chakra before me is to connect joyfully to All That Is, and to know that I am a co-creator.

Progressing linearly up the south ridge brings us to the area of the brow chakra, which is a mile-long ridge above the Featherbed. The heart and third chakra are no longer visible, blocked by the chin. The view to the east, west, and south is a meditative experience. It is so expansive and magnificent, especially when the sun is glistening on the water, that it stops you in your tracks. Having an endless view over the water to the east and south (respectively representing new beginnings and the direction closest to spirit on the medicine wheel) seems to open doors in my consciousness that I normally keep closed. Up here I feel alive.

As we leave the brow chakra to go to the crown, the trail descends into a wooded valley. I had always felt uneasy on this section of the trail, so one day I asked why. I was told that this was literally and symbolically the final dip before reaching the top—the last descent into darkness before reaching the light, so to speak.

At the top there are two peaks. One is set up for tourists with a trail and signs; the other is where I called to the spirit of the Mountain. This is where the trail brings you. There was a hotel here at one time. You see remnants of bricks and occasionally a square nail. Most people stay on the other knoll, so if your inclinations are towards connecting with the Mountain, it is possible to have time alone here. It can also be done anywhere.

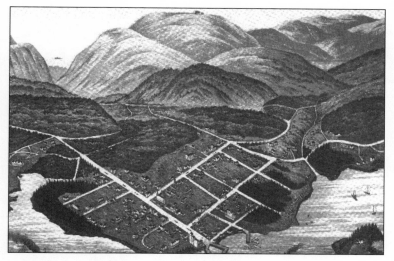

A bird's-eye-view of Bar Harbor, Maine.

In closing I want to summarize the salient points in this book. A transition is occurring. We are becoming conscious of the totality of ourselves, unifying all of our lifetimes into the present. Unification means resolving all unresolved lifetimes because they impact the present; clearing the subconscious of limiting programs because the low self is the link between the conscious self and our high self or spirit; and bringing our male and female sides, the will and the heart, into balance.

The low self, the Earth, and all of nature interconnect and communicate at the theta brainwave. The theta brainwave is our dream state; communication is symbolic, not literal. In theta we are one with spirit. Therefore, the

Earth and nature are actually spirit constantly communicating symbolically. This symbolic communication especially makes itself known at power spots on the Earth.

Imbalances in the low self correspond to imbalances in our chakras. Psychological and emotional issues determine which chakras are affected. Spending time at the chakra centers on the Earth, like the ones on Mount Desert Island, acts to balance the chakra centers of the body.

Mount Desert Island has a lot of heart. It facilitates our connection to our high self, which opens the channels for resolving unresolved lifetimes. Our feelings are pipelines to other dimensions and lifetimes. Walking and sitting on the Earth, the "breath to heart" technique, the "fox walk" with wide-angle vision, shamanic journeys, and vision quests are a few techniques that can facilitate balance.

From my heart to yours, I wish you clarity and success in your own quest for unity with all there is.